ASTHMA AND EMOTION

ASTHMA
and
EMOTION

by

Abraham Stern, Ph.D.

GARDNER PRESS, INC.
New York

Gardner Press, Inc.
19 Union Square West
New York 10003

Library of Congress Cataloging in Publication Data

Stern, Abraham, Ph.D.
   Asthma and emotion.

   Bibliography: p.
   Includes index.
   1. Asthma—Psychological aspects. 2. Emotions.
I. Title. [DNLM: 1. Asthma—Psychology. 2. Asthma
—Therapy. 3. Group processes. 4. Psychotherapy,
Group. 5. Emotions. WF 533 S839a]
RC591.S74   616.2'38   81-2383
ISBN 0-89876-002-X   AACR2

Printed in the United States of America

CONTENTS

To MMHS

Many women have done valiantly, but you excel them all . . .

Prov. 31:29

PREFACE

Conservative estimates indicate that 8.9 million Americans suffer from asthma. This figure does not count people who have had reactions in the past, but have since recovered. Of all Americans living today about fifteen million have had, have, or will have asthma.[1] The illness is particularly devasting to the young, with asthma the leading cause of school absence resulting from illness.[2]

This book is an attempt at a new approach to asthma treatment and rehabilitation. Though aspects of it may prove useful to all asthma sufferers, it is aimed particularly at the 10 to 12 percent of asthmatics whose ailment is considered to be "intractable"; that is, those who respond minimally, or not at all, to treatment. It is our contention that much can be done to improve their condition.

The pages that follow are dedicated to helping this large group of sufferers, both children and adults, to better understand their illness; to show them how others have been aided; and to suggest what they can do to help themselves or a loved one in their family who is an asthmatic.

INTRODUCTION

By training I am a social group worker.

For the first twenty years after I graduated from social work school, I was engaged in practice, primarily with vigorous boys, girls, men, and women, in a range of group settings: Y's, community centers, settlement houses, camps, national youth organizations, and at a university youth service bureau. Simultaneously I served as Associate Professor instructing in Social Work at Yeshiva University. The focus of my work during this entire period was on group services, and I dealt mostly with physically healthy people within all these settings.

From both theoretical and practical vantage points, it was apparent to me throughout this time that the small social group was unique in that it contained within itself the capacity and capability to serve as both the *setting* and the *medium* for effectuating individual movement. In other words, the social group workers' "group" could be seen as both the context and the tool for achieving better functioning of people by fostering growth and bringing about change. Not only social group workers, but progressive educators, therapists, and others whose work calls for them to utilize small groups, have likewise come to appreciate the significant potential for social change inherent in the small group. What is particularly striking is the dynamics—the subtle pressures, the encouragement and support that the group appears to possess—which can energize and effectuate wide-ranging change in personality, attitude, and conduct.

The evolution during the past decade or so of the use of the small group as an agent of "remediation" and "rehabilitation,"[3] in addition to its function as a socialization medium, became more fully meaningful to me a few years ago, when I spent a sabbatical abroad, serving as senior lecturer at the School of Social Work of the Bar Ilan University in Ramat Gan, Israel.

In this pulsating, new academic setting, faculty members were encouraged to undertake "demonstration projects" in an attempt to relate theoretical classroom instructional skills to real-life situations beyond the ivory towers of academia, and to thus broaden the base of social work practice, knowledge, and awareness in the country. The setting which I selected was Tel Aviv's Hadassa (Municipal) Hospital. The assignment was to introduce group work services to try to demonstrate how the small group could become a useful medium for the restoration of patients' physical and emotional well-being.

I was fortunate to have with me a unit of eight alert, sensitive, and capable upper classmen from the school, who would be assisting in the demonstration project, while simultaneously utilizing the setting for their clinical field-work training.

In retrospect, I can now all the more appreciate the courage and daring of the Hospital administration and staff in providing us the opportunity to break ground and in encouraging the initiation of creative efforts in several of its departments.

It was with a combination of anticipation and apprehension that the team was received by the hospital staff. Notwithstanding their excellent training at the School of Social Work, the students, in the best traditions of medicine, were not allowed to approach patients until they had undergone a thorough orientation by department heads and medical specialists on the etiology, manifestation, and symptoms of disease and illness. In addition, the hospital's chief psychiatrist offered his input on the psychological components of sickness.

Most of them European in origin, Hadassa's physicians had been trained to focus on the physical aspects of illness—an area in which they displayed considerable competence. In the main they were cordial but understandably guarded about the new process, and the implications for their patients and departments, of an approach which, in an effort to support treatment goals, sought to identify behavior that seemed to exacerbate a particular condition, and to work toward change in order to prevent a recurrence of symptomology.

In some of the Hospital departments—i.e., children's, rehabilitation, and renal dialysis (nephrology)—where the significance of the psychological component was more apparent, an understanding of our method came more easily to the medical staff than it did in others, such as internal medicine or the oncology sections, where it was less clearly perceived.

It was a slow, and at times trying experience to attempt to interpret to hard-headed, physically oriented physicians, that an opportunity for patients to function in a small social system, to share apprehensions, to receive reassurance and support from each other and from a worker, could be an important and meaningful process on their road to recovery. It took some interpretation to convince them that the physical condition of the post-coronary patient—whose concern, through group participation, was moving away from a preoccupation with the beeps of his EKG monitor toward greater self-awareness, and possible resolution of some of his inner strife and turmoil related to anxiety over family, job, or housing—was actually being helped in some way. But *how?* the physicians insisted on knowing.

Was it significant, they questioned, that an oncology patient who for months had been wrapped up in her illness to the exclusion of all else, but who was gradually displaying a little more concern for her appearance, combing her hair and applying make-up, as well as talking about life, current events, the theater, and displaying an interest in her family and in others rather than being preoccupied with death—did this really mean anything? Did it in any way change the course of her condition?

This question was repeated many times.

Our involvement with the Hospital's allergy clinic initially began as a result of our desire to give students an opportunity to work with "long-term patient groups," comprised preferably of youngsters, in which they might be able to observe various stages of group development, something akin to that which they might later experience in the more conventional work settings outside of the Hospital. These might include veteran's homes, community centers, Y's, or geriatric settings, where association with the same clients would continue for a period of a year or longer, rather than for merely a "short term." Since the average duration of a patient's stay in pediatrics, or internal medicine, for example, was approximately 10 to 12 days, for a solid learning experience we gravitated toward patients who might have a more extended association with the Hospital.

Our involvement with the out-patient asthmatic youngsters was a natural one. There was a large population of out-patient intractable asthmatics, in the main young, who had unfortunately had a rather lengthy association with the Hospital, and, given the nature of the illness, the outlook was that this association would in all likelihood be sustained. Further, the director of the Hospital's Asthma Clinic was interested in trying out our "new" approach.

Though this was our original motivation in seeking to work with asthma patients, the results of our quest into this area were to prove rather startling.

Ultimately some of our students were assigned to several short-term patient groups in different departments of the Hospital, and others to long-term groups: renal dialysis, rehabilitation. Almost each student, however, was assigned to one or more out-patient groups of asthmatic children and their parents.

Asthma, as we were to discover, was one of the few medical conditions in which it was possible to clinically measure chronic airway resistance through spirometry (pulmonary function tests) and other means, and thus observe how a patient was progressing or responding to treatment.

After initial medical and psychological evaluation of candidates, our group programs got under way. Within several months, it became apparent through pulmonary testing and other critical indices—such as the amount of wheezing, and the frequency and intensity of attacks—that certain changes were taking place, which seemed to produce a reduction of asthmatic symptoms for most of the participating youngsters, a fact which even the hard-headed "physical" physicians began to notice. The doctors were curious as to what precipitated these changes, since other variables such as medication, treatment, and home life appeared to have remained fairly constant.

It was at this juncture that other Hospital department heads who had heard from the grapevine of our work with the asthma groups began to take a second look at the social group work process, and to become interested in exploring its potential for "remediation," "rehabilitation," and support of treatment goals, as well as for improved patient socialization, all of which now appeared to them to be possibly inherent in our method.

As the project with asthmatic youngsters continued, and the results of our early findings appeared to be reconfirmed, my interest in acquiring a more intensive knowledge about the ailment led me to undertake a study of the literature on asthma and other pulmonary illness. I received encouragement to continue to seek the application of group work principles toward identifying and changing patterns to prevent the recurrence of asthmatic symptoms from Dr. Nathan Lass, Director of Hadassa's Allergy Clinic, from the late Dr. Donald Adler, Head of the Pediatric Allergy Department of the Mount Sinai Hospital in New York, from Dr. David Stein of the Brooklyn Jewish Hospital, from Dr. Elliot Middleton and Dr. Chaim Chai of the Children's Asthmatic Research Institute of Denver, from Dr. Murray Peshkin, Dean of America's allergists, from Dr. Harold Abramson, Editor of the *Journal of Asthma Research*, and from Dr. Larry Ross of the Albert Einstein College of Medicine. Their support led me to believe that the Bar-Ilan-Hadassa experimental project had something to say to asthma sufferers not only in Israel, but elsewhere.

Their inspiration also helped add a new dimension to my own professional career and stimulated a desire to share some of our Hadassa findings. We did so first at the International Obstructive Lung Disease Conference in Haifa, then at the International Pediatric Conference in Jerusalem, and later at various medical and psychological meetings in the United States.

It was the encouragement received from these men which led me to further study, exploration, and practice, and ultimately to the preparation of this book, to demonstrate the value of treatment of the intractable asthmatic through the medium of the small social group.

ASTHMA AND
EMOTION

1

WHAT IS ASTHMA?

How Do We Breathe?

The breathing or respiratory equipment in man looks like an upside-down tree. Originating from the middle of the chest, the trachea, a trunklike tube, separates to create two bronchi, one leading to each lung. The bronchi in turn divide into smaller bronchi, which spread out like leaves into numerous small bronchioles, each leading into tiny balloon-like air sacs called alveoli. The lung tissue is made up of these alveoli wrapped tightly in small blood vessels which cover the bronchial tubes.

In the process of breathing, air enters and leaves the lungs, which react like a sponge. When squeezed, the alveoli, the tiny air cells, force out carbon dioxide. When the pressure is released, they expand, the tiny cells filling with air rich in oxygen. The oxygen is removed from the air in the lungs through the thin-walled blood vessels surrounding the alveoli, and is replaced with carbon dioxide.

The entire bronchial tract is lined with a smooth membrane whose glands secrete a mucus which acts as a lubricant, to facilitate the passage of air through the tubes. The walls of the bronchi are elastic and enable contraction and expansion during the process of respiration.

What Is Asthma?

When asthma occurs, there is a constriction of the muscles of the bronchial walls, which reduces the flow of air to the small air sacs. A slight muscular contraction of the bronchial wall can cause constriction and interference in normal respiration.

During an attack of asthma, the membrane of the tiny bronchial tubes swells. The obstruction prevents or impedes the flow of air and the normal emptying of the alveoli, which remain hyperinflated, or stretched to capacity, with air. An excess of mucus is produced and secreted. It accumulates in the bronchial tubes, hardening as it dries, and becomes thick and viscous, thus further reducing the flow of air. As this occurs the air is trapped in the lungs, and the individual experiences shortness of breath, often accompanied by a feeling of tightness in the chest, dyspnea (an air hunger), a choking sensation and a coughing spasm which is an effort of the airways to remove the obstruction.

Wheezing

Wheezing occurs as a result of the bronchial constriction, and is often accompanied by a dry cough and by sputum.

A mild asthma attack can generally be relieved if the sputum, which usually resembles small beads, can be coughed up. When the air cannot be removed from the lungs, a reduction in the amount of oxygen reaching the bloodstream results. In severe, chronic cases, the number of red blood cells in the blood increases, with a concomitant decrease of the oxygen supply to the body tissues. The resulting change in the acid-base balance in the system can lead to damage to the lungs and heart.

Severity of Attacks

A bronchial asthma attack may take place occasionally or with regularity, and may be mild, severe, life threatening, and sometimes even fatal. Symptoms may vary from a heaviness on the chest to "status asthma," which is intense and persistent asthma caused by the bronchial tubes going into spasm, which can induce unconsciousness and cause significant changes in the chemistry and metabolism of the body.

A concern over frequent attacks is that air trapped in the alveoli, the small sacs, can cause the lungs to remain permanently inflated. In this extreme condition, the alveoli may lose their elasticity and break or tear, with a number of the sacs fusing, or becoming one. If this happens often, a more limited surface is created, so that air that cannot be exhaled remains permanently trapped in the inflated alveoli. Normal inspiration and expiration are thus inhibited, and an increased amount of stagnant air is left behind with expiration. If this situation persists and is untreated, it may lead to the onset of a condition in which the air sac walls lose their elasticity, and with it their capability to expand and contract, to inspire and to expire.

Many youngsters who have suffered from asthma since infancy outgrow their condition. Some develop it later in life. For some, asthma attacks occur with moderate frequency and severity, and there are long periods of freedom from symptoms. For others, being asthmatic can mean being perpetually out of breath. Such sufferers begin to wheeze quickly in response to various stimuli.

The inability to breathe can be a frightening experience. An attack that comes with little advance warning may create a state of panic, which can accentuate the breathing difficulty.

A Complicated Illness

The description offered above is perhaps an over-simplification of a complex illness. Extensive research has fairly well established that asthma is a complicated illness which is related to the functioning of the central nervous system and to immunological disorders. It has also become increasingly apparent that asthma is affected by allergies and infections as well as by emotional and psychological factors. These influences vary from case to case, and may exist by themselves, or in association with each other.

The Role of Allergens

The allergic person's body is sensitive to invasion by foreign substances. While the nonallergic person can breathe fresh air freely, the person allergic to pollen in the air may sneeze, cough, wheeze, or otherwise feel distressed if there is even a slight amount of pollen present.

In this instance the offending substance is pollen, but an allergen or antigen can be almost any foreign substance that offends enough to cause an allergic reaction.

Allergens or antigens are most often stopped from entering the body by our first line of defense, our skin, or by the membrane which covers our breathing and digestive tracts. Usually the first exposure to an allergen produces sensitization, with the second or third exposure causing a "reaction." In some instances sensitization occurs before birth.

We should be aware that it is possible for people to develop sensitivity not only to outside allergens but also to the bacteria which they harbor in their own body. This is especially true for bacteria which are found in the nose, tonsils, throat, bronchi, ears, and sinuses. It is because of this "bacteria allergy" that there is a frequent association of allergy in infectious diseases, such as in attacks of asthma following respiratory infection. Viruses, parasites, and other infectious agents may also produce allergies.

Currently there are felt to be two extremes in so called allergic or "intrinsic" asthma versus so called "infective" or "extrinsic" asthma. The exact role of allergy in relation to clinical asthma remains speculative though there are numerous examples of asthmatics with highly allergic diathesis [susceptibility]. Further bronchospasm is a final common pathway of both asthma and many allergic responses.[4]

How One Becomes Allergic

If foreign protein is able to get beyond our natural barriers—our skin and the membrane which covers our respiratory and digestive tracts—the body is usually able to get rid of it through the lungs, the kidneys, or the intestines.

Allergy represents an atopic (hyper-sensitive) reaction to foreign protein which has penetrated the first line defense (stem or mucus membrane). In those people with an allergic tendency, such foreign proteins can evoke the formation of reaginic antibodies (Immuno Globulin E). These antibodies combine specifically with the allergen and liberate or cause the release of secondary mediators of inflammation such as histamines and other vasoactive peptides. The response in the lung consists of excessive mucus production and bronchospasm.

Thus, if a foreign protein is able to get past the body's defenses, it is possible for one to become allergic. If a person suffers from repeated colds, for example, the frequent irritation of the mucus membrane in the nose, windpipe, and bronchial tubes helps to create a series of symptoms: stuffy nose, sneezing, wheezing, coughing, expectorating, shortness of breath, and other manifestations of "allergy of the respiratory tract" to which hay fever, bronchitis, and asthma are related.

Some of the more common offending allergens are:[5]

Inhaled substances, including pollens from trees, weeds, grasses, and plants; dust; mold spores.
Animal dander (skin or hair shed from animals). This may include fur or clothing such as rabbit collars and fur-lined gloves; also pets and feathers.
Foods such as shellfish, lobster, crab, fish, chocolate, nuts, spices, eggs, milk, wheat, certain fruits and vegetables.
Substances which come into contact with the skin: plastics, metals,

rubber, fabrics, dyes, cosmetics, resin, drugs, hand lotions, insecticides, sprays, foliage, or certain plants (poison ivy, for example).

Drugs: Those given by injection, such as antibiotics, serums, hormones, liver extracts, and insulin; and those taken by mouth including aspirin, laxatives, sedatives, sleeping pills, and tranquilizers.

2
PHYSICAL, PSYCHOLOGICAL, OR HEREDITARY?

Do the facts support the contention that asthma is heredi tary, or is asthma primarily a physical, or psychological condition?

Research has shown that 60 percent of asthmatics have a history of allergy in their family, while fewer than 7 percent of nonasthmatics have allergic antecedents.[6] Are these figures not sufficient proof that genetic factors play a vital role in this illness? Does it not appear likely that there is a predisposition, an inherent structural or constitutional weakness among asthmatics, or that an innate sensitivity may exist in the asthmatic's breathing apparatus which relates back to birth? Is it not possible that one comes into this world with a vulnerable respiratory tract which reacts to stimuli, possibly the antigen-antibody mechanism?

Though many physicians and researchers are prepared to accept the statistical data—the discrepancy between the 60 percent and the 7 percent figures—as conclusive evidence that the condition is largely hereditary, the behaviorists have their own interpretation of these figures.

While they recognize the important role of genetics, structural factors, and vulnerability, they view the heavy incidence of asthma running through families as indications of the presence in these families of unique psychological and emotional attitudes and traits which appear to be transferred from mother to child. They believe that there may be a syndrome within the organization and functioning of the asthmatics' family constellations of intrapsychic and interpersonal factors which may be perpetuating the chronicity of the illness.

If this assumption is accurate, it may also help us to understand the manifestation of the so-called "neurotic behavior" of the asthmatic.

Cause and Effect in Asthma

To the careful observer, the asthmatic's behavior often appears strange, perhaps even somewhat neurotic. A multitude of adjectives has been used to describe him. These include, among others, denying, overcompensating, depressed, embarrassed, and lacking in confidence. Assuming for argument's sake that these descriptions are accurate, and that neurotic manifestations are present, the question which arises is: are the factors associated with this neurotic behavior in response to the asthma symptoms, or are they caused by the symptoms? For example, can the asthmatic's frequent utilization of denial and overcompensation, which are seen as aspects of his "maladjustment," possibly be viewed as "defenses" against the debilitating features of his illness, or can the asthmatic's depression be the result of his inability to control his condition even through medication? Isn't it reasonable to assume that the facial disfigurement brought on by prolonged use of corticosteroids will lead to embarrassment over one's appearance? Would a patient's refusal in this instance to continue his medication, result in the development of additional symptoms?

Other related questions which we should consider, are: How does the patient who is often viewed by others as sick or weak, come to view himself? How does his negative image of himself, and his limited self-confidence, relate to his illness?

What of the child who has limited contact with his peers because of a number of restrictions, or whose relations with siblings has deteriorated because he has been treated differently than they: is his behavioral maladjustment due to his condition or to limitations in his functioning?

Do the exacerbated feelings of parents who are wrapped up in frustration, resentment, and self-blame over their child's condition contribute to their child's feelings?

In other words, is it really possible in such cases to separate responses to symptoms from responses caused by symptoms?

In an effort to respond to some of these questions, the allergist Aaron Lask says: "It is playing with words to ask if such [emotional] illness causes asthma, or is an effect of it." He continues,

We found that severely ill asthmatics who do not respond to routine treatment *usually have grave emotional illness, sometimes but not always, at the conscious level. It is playing with words to ask if such illness causes asthma, or is an effect of it.* What is clear, is that successful resolution of the emotional difficulties leads to the virtual disappearance of asthma, and failure to resolve the problem is associated with the persistence of the asthma. Those physicians who do not *find emotional conflict* in status asthmatics [read chronic intractable asthmatics] are so to speak, emotionally tone deaf.[7]

To Dr. Lask there seems to be little doubt that emotional factors are inextricably bound up with asthma. If he is right, then it is an almost pointless exercise to speculate on the separation of cause and effect. Instead we might focus on the fact that a chronic illness is the major variable, and as such, it should not surprise us that there appears to be a greater amount of behavior disturbance in asthmatics and their families than in the nonasthmatic population.

Psychological Makeup of Asthmatics

What have the researchers identified as the unique psychological characteristics of the asthmatic? Most interestingly, there does not appear to be any single type of asthma personality. Instead of a homogeneous profile, we find a great amount of heterogeneity in a psychological composite of an asthmatic. Here's what some of the researchers found:

Asthmatics possessed feelings of persecution and a strong fear of death.[8]

They were inhibitive in demonstrating anger, and in their self-assertion.[9]

Asthmatic children seem to set higher goals for themselves than do healthy children.[10]

Though they often displayed high intelligence in verbal tests, they had poor performance ability. They were over-anxious, and limited in self-confidence.[11]

The Families of Asthmatic Children

A significant amount of neurotic behavior was also found to be present in the families of asthmatic youngsters. A high incidence of psychoneurosis appeared to exist among relatives of asthmatics,[12] and more than half of asthmatics surveyed in one study had one or more near relatives with either psychoneurosis or psychosis.[13]

The Special Relationship of the Asthmatic and His Parents

The close emotional involvement between the asthmatic child and his or her mother is cited repeatedly by researchers. While generalizations may have little bearing on specific cases, the volume of literature bearing on the special relationship of the asthmatic child and his parents, particularly concerning that between mother and child, is exceedingly large. A sample of some of the thinking follows.

High, Often Unattainable Goals. The asthmatic children's feelings of insecurity are reinforced by the higher goals that their mothers set for them—goals which they were often unable to attain.[14]

= love

Alternating Between Seduction, Over-concern, and Rejection. Asthmatic children see their mothers as alternating between extremes of seduction, over-concern, and intolerant rejection. The children show strong but ambivalent ties to their mothers, and unconsciously fear them.[15]

Overdependence and Control. The asthmatic child appears to be over-dependent upon his mother, and he is valued by her only when he is sick. The child's asthma attacks may be in compliance with the mother's unconscious desire to control the child, the reasoning being that when he is ill, the child shows how dependent he is on his mother; and when this happens, he is gratifying her wishes.[16]

Conflict Over Separation and Dependency. The disturbed mother-child relationship has received considerable attention by researchers. The mothers of asthmatics often tend to have ambivalent attitudes toward their children. They are over-protective, and seek to bind the child in a dependent situation. The asthmatic attack is seen by another researcher as an expression of opposing tendencies: a protest against the separation from the mother, and a protest against wanting to establish a dependent relationship with the mother.[17]

Hostility Turned Inward. Some believe that the allergic child is unable to express his hostility toward his parents. He tries to repress it, but repression only partially relieves his inner tensions. When this happens, "the child turns his own body into the target of his anger."[18] By discharging the hostility toward himself, the child punishes himself for the feelings he would ordinarily be too afraid to admit to his consciousness.

Children Born at an Inopportune Time. In a study of 20 mothers of asthmatic children aged 5 to 12, it was found that many mothers felt that their child had come into their lives at an "inopportune time." On the whole, the mothers appeared to be rather ineffective in handling their children. Asthma served as a means for the children to demand more attention, which in turn stimulated dependent, clinging behavior. "Asthma," the researchers suggested, "may be called a disease of dependency."[19]

Confusion Over Role. It was observed in the course of group psychotherapy sessions with the parents of asthmatic children that many felt confused about the concept of their role as parent.[20]

Reliving Patterns. Parents appeared to relive in their children the patterns of their own childhood.[21]

Conflict Over Anxiety, Guilt and Adequacy. In another study, mothers of asthmatic children were found to have conflicting feelings both about their children and their own roles as mothers. They felt anxious and guilty toward their children and inadequate as mothers.

The Cronus Complex. The unique Cronus Complex, involving "mutual engulfment," was seen as operating between mother and child. The parent, according to this theory, has preconceived notions of what the child should be like. An emotionally immature parent who finds it difficult to deal with a growing child, seeks to coerce him into a pattern structured upon the parent's own immaturity. The child, who is handicapped by both illness and a narcissistic mother, is "forced during development into a distorted state of dependency."[22]

The growing child is seen as conflicted by his need to develop independence and maturity, while being constantly threatened by controlling parents. The engulfing parent manipulates every act of the child. Rejection may arise when the mutual engulfment fails to satisfy the parental needs.

Common Features of Theories

The list of theories I have presented, though by no means complete, is representative of those concerning the unique parental, and particularly the mother-child, relationship of the asthmatic. Upon closer examination, several recurrent themes predominate:

1. There is confusion, anxiety, and guilt related to the mother's feelings of inadequacy in her role.
2. There is conflict on the part of the mother over the child's struggle for increased independence.
3. There is manipulation of the child to comply with, and

gratify, the mother's narcissistic or neurotic needs.
4. Throughout, there is repeated rejection, repression, and hostility, over-protection, over-concern, and over-dependence.

If we are to ascribe validity to these findings, we are faced with the need to reconcile obviously disparate behavior forms. How do we square feelings of rejection and over-protection, repression, and over-concern? Aren't these conflicting manifestations?

Different Forms of Rejection

The apparent disparity may be reconciled if we introduce a definition of rejection which covers most of the theories presented. Three forms of rejection, are identified, the most obvious being overt hostility. In this case, the parent, under the guise of "corrective effort," nags, threatens, and otherwise manifests cruelty toward his child.

A second form of parental rejection is perfectionism. The assertion here is that the child cannot be loved as he is, but if he improves, the situation might be different.

A third form of rejection is compensatory overprotection; the prevailing attitude being: "No one can possibly find a flaw in the mother's conduct, since so much is being given up, and all pleasures are being denied for the benefit of the child."[23]

According to this view the parent may be playing out a single form, or a combination of rejection modalities simultaneously.

Impact on the Child

As a result of this type of parental behavior toward him, the child too alternates between hating his hostile parent and feeling guilty for this hatred, because after all, the overprotecting parent is denying himself so much for the child's benefit. In each instance, the child is not in total control of the consequences. He is often unable to achieve and is never able to fully satisfy his parents while maintaining his individuality.

We thus see the asthmatic child as terribly conflicted. No matter how hard he tries to please, he can rarely satisfy the complex needs of parents, who unbeknown to him are often subtly manipulating him to fulfill their own repressed desires.

His frustration gives rise to feelings of anger, fear, resentment, and anxiety, which in turn affect his condition, as we shall see in the next chapter.

(1) the child is trying to achieve individuality and independence.

(2) Insecure attachment.

(3) child serves parent rather than parent serving child

3

THE ROLE OF ANGER, FEAR, ANXIETY, AND STRESS

Man as a vital, active, and creative being, is surrounded almost constantly by emotionally challenging situations. These challenges take on a variety of forms, at times appearing as threats to man's physical self or to his survival as a person. At other times these challenges are perceived as threats which endanger his personality, as when a person is faced with the loss of love, prestige, security, or status.

Since so many people are out of touch with their feelings, emotions are often undifferentiated, and go unrecognized. People's real feelings rarely come to the surface as they are, but are rather expressed in disguised forms. To illustrate, tension may really conceal feelings of fear, hurt feelings may serve as a cover-up for anger, tears and an inability to concentrate may be a disguise for moodiness, and resentment, a mask for depression.

Concealment of Real Feelings

Most people tend to repress their feelings rather than face them on a conscious level. Many may not even be aware of their feelings, probably because it is considered a sign of weakness in our society to display emotions. The individual who is unable or unwilling to express his emotions, substitutes for his real feelings responses which he believes are more socially acceptable.

Society's depersonalization of people is a major factor contributing to man's inability to express his true feelings. The organization and structure of our contemporary world and the pace of modern life encourage man to conceal, rather than to reveal, himself. Friendliness and human association, which may lead to openness, are rare commodities. For example the local storekeeper, who at one time provided an opportunity for personal contact, has been replaced by the impersonal supermarket cashier. Apartment-house and development dwellers consider anonymity preferable to neighborliness. The comfort, identity, and sense of sharing which were provided in the past by the extended family, have with the demise of that institution virtually disappeared. What was formerly the ultimate sanctuary, man's home, has been rocked by changes in life styles which have brought reductions in opportunities for communication and conversation in which people could share their real feelings.

It makes little difference whether emotional hurts are experienced on a conscious level, whether they are disguised, denied, or considered nonexistent, since their effect is similar. These can even occur when a person is unaware of the existence within him of feelings of anger or resentment, or when one merely recalls an angry experience. As a matter of fact, the recollection of an insult or a threat may provoke anger or resentment so intense that at times it even outweighs the feelings of an actual experience. A challenge to a person's ego can likewise provoke a response as severe as if he were being physically threatened. When a person's feelings are hurt repeatedly, or when he anticipates being hurt, feelings of anger and resentment which ultimately lead to feelings of being "threatened" often develop.

As far as the consequences are concerned, almost all emotionally threatening experiences can be harmful if repeated with sufficient frequency or intensity.

Individual Differences

People vary in the degree of their arousal to frustration and anger. The reason for these differences is not overly clear, nor do we fully understand why some individuals are more emotionally reactive than others. Resentment may bring out feelings of helpless indignation that have been bottled up over long periods of time. It is conceivable too that some people are more sensitive because of unhappy experiences which they may have sustained in their childhood, or because they are carrying a heavy load of undischarged anger.

Anger and Fear

Attempts have been made to draw a distinction between anger and fear, though the effects of both can be quite disturbing and harmful. The distinction is seen as follows: in the case of anger, the event or condition that arouses the anger is usually in the past, while fear involves the apprehension of an event or condition which may occur. If viewed this way, fear and anger become part of a sequence, yet as one behaviorist observed, the "threat of harm can be a harm in itself, by disturbing a man's peace of mind and arousing fear."[24]

Thus fear may result from the presence or threat of an actual harm or danger. The danger or threat may be to a person's life, his ego, his health, his possessions, his security, his virility, his beliefs, or to his self-esteem.

Just as people tend to conceal their true feelings in other areas, they may, for a variety of reasons, also be unable to express their feelings of anger or fear. Their inability may be predicated upon a reluctance to risk being rejected or abandoned. Their reluctance to express anger or fear may also be because they feel unworthy, or because they have a need to punish themselves. When anger or fear cannot be expressed or displaced appropriately, it is frequently turned inward and can harm the person who is experiencing that feeling.

What often influences or determines the extent of the harm a threat or fear may do is not so much the anticipation of the experience, as the person's own sense of adequacy—how capable he feels of coping with the particular situation. For example, if he feels capable of coping, he may become angry; if, however, he feels inadequate, he is more likely to become frightened.

The precipitants of fear need not be only dramatic threats to life, but they can be common, almost every-day occurrences. People may be afraid of being disliked, or of being misunderstood. People are afraid of being bossed, or of being lonely, or disapproved of; or people may fear a loss of love, or that they will lose their power or prestige.

Fear of Self-Criticism

A person may be anxious or afraid of his own self-criticism, or of not living up to his ideals or to his code of behavior. The higher his standards, the more his conscience may bother him. Since his conscience is always telling him what to do, he may feel bound or unable to act on his own free will—conflicted between the need to obey his conscience and the fear of disobeying it.

Anxiety: Apprehension About an Unknown

While fear seems to be basically grounded in reality, apprehension about being hurt, mugged, or raped, about impending surgery, or losing a loved one—anxiety—generally refers to apprehension about an unknown.

Steincrohn has illustrated the difference between fear and anxiety as follows: "Fear occurs when you see an animal about to attack, or a plane about to crash. Anxiety is an ongoing or lasting tension." It has been described as a "low-grade persistent worry." "Should I take the plane although it might crash . . . ?" Anxiety has also been defined as "an impulse from within." Just as anger and fear from outside may induce apprehension, anxiety may also be precipitated by impulses from within. "Since anxiety is frequently continued over an extended period, its effects may be more pernicious . . . "[25]

The American Psychiatric Association's definition of anxiety is "apprehension, tension, or uneasiness which stems from anticipation of danger, the source of which is largely unknown or unrecognized."

Because the source of anxiety is often unknown, or the person is unaware of the reasons for his anxiety, it becomes all the more difficult to handle. Once it is identified, though, and becomes a specific fear, it is then an emotion which lends itself to being handled.

Fear of Domination

A particularly strong fear, one that appears to be present in people for months and often years, is the fear of domination, which entails the loss of personality and free will. Domination, or removal of one's ability to decide things for oneself, may come about either because one has constantly been told what to do, or because one has been smothered by so many good suggestions that one does not have the power to choose an alternative.

The individual whose loved ones dominate him has to do what they (usually his parents or spouse) want him to do. He is afraid that if he does not perform according to their wishes, they will be disapproving or their feelings hurt. In his efforts to comply and to do what they expect or want him to do, he fears that he is becoming a part of another's personality, and is losing his capacity to have wants of his own, or to have an independent existence. This apprehension is sometimes accompanied by an almost paralyzing feeling of inadequacy or general helplessness. It can result in a person's inability to handle the challenges of every-day life, and may lead to a state of constant apprehension and worry. Since the individual is not necessarily aware of the cause of this fear, its very nonspecificity makes it even more awesome than it is. He is afraid without knowing why. Since the cause of his fear is unknown, speculation of the cause may precipitate even further apprehension.[26]

A child may feel strong anxiety in the presence of a parent or another person whom he does not want to hurt. If he is angry at his parents but is unable to show it or talk about his feelings because he might lose their love, or because they might be angered and punish him, acute anxiety may be aroused. As stated, a particular danger is that feelings of anger which cannot be expressed are often directed inward, to the person himself, causing him to hurt himself as a means of making the overly dominating parent feel guilty.

Stress

What is stress?

To most people stress implies a type of emotional arousal—fear or anxiety, or a form of physical exertion. Stressful events may affect people differently even when caused by the same stimulus, so it is important to evaluate not only stressful situations, but also how a particular person responds to the occurrence.

In the psychological sense, stress generally refers to situations which people see as threatening to them. Up to a certain level, people have a remarkable capacity to adapt. When their tolerance level or threshold has been surpassed, the emotional change begins to set physiological change into motion.

Threatening, stress-producing situations affect people at different stages of their life, and are not limited to a particular age or period of development. For an adult, it may be an impending marital crisis, serious illness, or the loss of a job. A youngster may feel threatened by the rejection of parents or friends, by feelings of inadequacy, or by an inability to measure up to his own expectations or to those which someone else has established for him.

Just as in the case of anger, fear, and anxiety, when we assess stress potential, consideration must be given to the specific tolerance level of the individual. For some, even too much pleasant stimulation may prove stressful, the pleasant stimulation taxing the body's ability to respond normally. Therefore pleasing but demanding events such as a long swim, or remaining up for an all-night party, may for some prove to be more than their body is able to cope with.

As we have indicated for other emotional challenges, in order for stress to be felt, the particular offending event does not even have to take place. It is sufficient for the situation merely to be perceived as threatening. Even a potential failure in the mind of the beholder—for example, an individual's concern about whether he will be able to make new friends, or be accepted by colleagues on a new job is often sufficient to provoke a stressful response. So long as the possiblity of failure exists, one can be under stress.

The intensity of the anticipated perception, or of a particular concern or situation, will vary to the extent of failure anticipated by the given threat, the conditioning, past experiences, the person's image of himself, and related factors. The individual's ability to cope and the response to these factors will serve to determine the extent of the pyschological, and in turn the physiological influence on the body.

Effect on the Body

How is the body affected by stress?

Current thinking is that anxiety and stress are heavily related to a wide range of chronic illnesses. The effect of stress on health is considered as potentially more dangerous to man than many of the so-called harmful foods, polluted air, or the intake of tobacco. The British psychiatrist McGlashan observes in this regard that "anxiety, not tobacco or coffee or soft water, is the hidden destroyer of the contemporary world."[27]

Experimentation has shown that a variety of responses are produced by the autonomic nervous system, which in turn unconsciously creates physiological and biological changes in the body. The variable, as has been pointed out, is the individual's ability to cope. This ability may be based on physical and genetic factors in addition to the life experience and other individual social, and emotional capacities.

The noted stress researcher W. I. Thomas found that an individual's ability to come to terms with a given stress situation varied according to his "stress adjustment"—his ability on the basis of past situations to adjust to, meet, and master new situations. In other words, where sufficient stress experience has been gained in past encounters, these may well serve to relieve the intensity of the stress in similar occurrences in the future.[28]

Tension Residue

Anxiety and stress are viewed by Drs. Haugen, Dixon, and Dickel as "a learned physical reaction." These authors see anxiety building up in an individual during childhood and adolescence as a result of external or internal threats to his well-being. According to this theory, the body, which has tensed up in response to a threat, generally relaxes afterwards, though not completely; a degree of tension remains. When the threat reappears, the anxiety again causes the body to tense up. When the threat passes, there remains this time a larger residue of physical tension. Because the tension has not been completely discharged or brought to the surface, after repeated bouts with anxiety, the body, which continues to tense up each time, finds itself tensed up more permanently, although there may be less of a threat to account for the physical state of arousal.

According to this theory, the symptoms which begin to appear—digestive disorders, exaggerated heartbeat, insomnia, a continual headache, or in the cases presented here, asthmatic symptoms—are indications of anxiety. These symptoms have their origins in the psyche—the mind—but have become rooted in the body. In other words, when a part of the body is subjected to more stress than it can possibly cope with, or is kept in a state of continuous tension, that part of the body can lose its normal functioning capacity.[29]

There are several important implications to these findings, the most obvious being that people will respond differently to a given situation depending upon both constitutional and a variety of experiential and emotional factors. Not least of these is the ability to cope, to meet life's demands, which depends upon a person's preparation through familiarity and practice. Adaptation to, and recall of successful encounters reduces the apprehension and fear associated with the particular task or event when it occurs again.

To quote Thomas, "Given adequate preparatory activity, what under other circumstances may be highly threatening, causes little concern; the reactions are so routine that the complexity of the response usually goes unrecognized. Indeed, these coping responses become so habituated, that we often can do things more effectively than we can describe them."[30] The social community from which a person comes, his past experiences, his capabilities, and whether or not he wants to or can meet a particular challenge, are all relevant. All of these factors we can sum up in three attributes: 1) the individual's preparation for the challenge, 2) the incentives to meet it, and 3) the evaluating systems.

Change and Stress

Just as ongoing and continuous stress can have harmful effects on health, there is growing belief in the stress-producing potential of significant or multiple changes, be they undesirable or not. It appears from recent research that a number of radical changes occurring at a particular time can be especially devastating to health.

A study by Dr. Richard H. Rahe of 2,500 officers and enlisted men aboard three navy cruisers showed that men who had experienced the most significant amount of change (the system used to evaluate the amount of change achieved was a "life change score"; see Table 1) developed 90 percent more illness during their first month at sea than those who achieved the lowest life-change scores.[31] Rahe correlated the effect of life-style changes which had occurred during the preceding six months and the men's health during the next six months at sea. As the cruise continued, the increased ratio of illness among high-life-change scorers persisted. Indeed, there was a very close correlation between the two.

A similar study by Dr. Thomas Holmes, professor of psychiatry at the University of Washington, on the case histories of

5,000 civilian patients, likewise established that significant life-change situations appeared to occur in most instances shortly before the onset of major illness.[32]

The "cluster concept," which states that illness tends to take place around the time of major events and interactions of people with their environment—events which result in significant changes in one's life—has been demonstrated by a number of researchers. Holmes and Rahe's "Social Readjustment Rating Scale" represents an approximation of "amount, duration, and severity of change" required by a person to cope with a number of life events. Holmes and Rahe feel that the more changes a person experiences during a specific period of time (and the more intense the changes), the more stress points he will accumulate.

Table 1
Social Readjustment Rating Scale[a]

Rank	Life event	Mean value
1	Death of spouse	100
2	Divorce	73
3	Marital separation	65
4	Jail term	63
5	Death of close family member	63
6	Personal injury or illness	53
7	Marriage	50
8	Fired at work	47
9	Marital reconciliation	45
10	Retirement	45
11	Change in health of family member	44
12	Pregnancy	40
13	Sex difficulties	39
14	Gain of new family member	39
15	Business readjustment	39
16	Change in financial state	38
17	Death of close friend	37
18	Change to different line of work	36
19	Change in number of arguments with spouse	35
20	Mortgage over $10,000	31
21	Foreclosure of mortgage or loan	30
22	Change in responsibilities at work	29
23	Son or daughter leaving home	29
24	Trouble with in-laws	29

25	Outstanding personal achievement	28
26	Wife begin or stop work	26
27	Begin or end school	26
28	Change in living conditions	25
29	Revision of personal habits	24
30	Trouble with boss	23
31	Change in work hours or conditions	20
32	Change in residence	20
33	Change in schools	20
34	Change in recreation	19
35	Change in church activities	19
36	Change in social activities	18
37	Mortgage or loan less than $10,000	17
38	Change in sleeping habits	16
39	Change in number of family get-togethers	15
40	Change in eating habits	15
41	Vacation	13
42	Christmas	12
43	Minor violations of the law	11

[a]See Holmes, T. H., and Rahe, R. H. The Social Readjustment Rating Scale. *Journal of Psychosomatic Research 11*:213–218, 1967, for complete wording of the items. Reproduced by permission of the exclusive licensee for Pergamon back volumes. Microforms International Marketing Corporation.

An individual scoring below 150 points, they believe, is on pretty safe ground: there is a one in three chance of "serious health change in the next two years." A person whose score is between 150 and 300 points would see his chances rise to 50-50. If, however, the score is over 300 points, the chances of serious health change within the next two years, researchers feel, are almost 90 percent.

Holmes and his colleague Minoru emphasize that life-style changes do not have to be traumatic, such as the death of a mate, or divorce, to be stress inducing; but even an accumulation of every-day anxiety-producing episodes, such as family disagreements, or a child leaving home, can make for a highly significant correlation between life-change scores and chronic disease.[33]

While all of the above is highly relevant to the asthma-prone individual, an interesting corollary of the Holmes study is not to avoid change entirely, as many asthmatics are prone to do, but rather to avoid "too much change in too short a period of time."[34]

The impact of "life change," scientists seem to feel, can also be diminished if a person "can learn to regulate major changes that inevitably affect him."[35] If an individual can learn to regulate such change, he may simultaneously be developing a capability for defusing their consequences.

How emotional and psychological stress ultimately influence physical change in the asthmatic, perhaps more than in others, will be examined in the next chapter.

4

MIND AND BODY: HOW THEY INTERACT

The medical and psychological communities have come a long way toward resolving the question of whether organic illness creates emotional problems, or whether emotional problems precipitate and worsen organic illness.

The theory of psychosomatics attempts to resolve this conflict, pointing out that there is an intimate relationship between physical health and emotion, and that mind and body are inseparable. Emotional reactions, by stimulating changes in the body chemistry, induce physical changes, and correspondingly, physiological changes bring on emotional reactions. An individual's health therefore relates to his total being.[36]

The Autonomic Nervous System

Man's emotional response to his perception of things comes about in a section of the brain called the limbic system. A group of cells at the base of the brain, the hypothalamus, receive his impulses, and in turn proceed to activate the autonomic nervous system.

When an individual experiences strong emotional feelings, the endocrine balance can change as a result of the hormones which the hypothalamus secretes into the blood stream. This change can affect both blood supply and blood pressure. The chemical changes can likewise slow the process of digestion and cause changes in breathing.

The individual's physiological response can also cause tightening in the throat, heart palpitations, and cold sweat. Changes in breathing and body temperature may occur. The continued pressure of strong emotional factors can cause a change in the output of the glands and in the release of hormones. Overproduction of hormones may, if sustained, bring on changes which can lead to illness.

Why These Changes Occur

For the body to function properly, and for the individual to remain healthy, it is necessary for the "body environment"—the heart rate, blood pressure, oxygen level, and amount of nutrients in the blood—to maintain a measure of constancy. Changes in this balance can result from intense emotions, germs, injury, inadequate air supply, or from a breakdown of parts of the body due to aging.

Since the body cannot tolerate drastic changes, when change threatens to go too far, a number of minor adjustments occur in the system to prevent the original change from overpowering the body.

Harvard physiologist Dr. Walter B. Cannon calls the system's ability to confront sudden life-threatening situations, the "wisdom of the body."[37] Cannon found that when the human organism is suddenly faced with intense danger or fear, a significant amount of adrenaline pours into its bloodstream. The sympathetic nervous system, in response to an intense nervous reaction, releases an almost identical hormone, noradrenaline.

These changes in the body improve the likelihood of survival: as circulation speeds up, more energy-rich sugar appears in the blood. The blood clotting mechanism is accelerated, muscle functioning is strengthened, and breathing is speeded up. The release into circulation of blood cells previously in storage, contributes to a sharper functioning of the senses.

The paleness and chilliness following injury or shock, are brought about by changes in the circulation, which attempt to assure that the heart and brain will receive a sufficient supply of blood to respond to the new condition. The body, Dr. Cannon notes, is thus prepared for "fight or flight."

Dr. Hans Selye of the University of Montreal researched thousands of medical cases in an effort to understand how the body reacts to various types of injury, disease, poison, excessive stimulation, or work demand.[38] He found similarities and common features in almost each case studied, regardless of the nature of the disease or injury. In his classic work, *The Stress of Life,* Dr. Selye, after separating out change features unique to a specific condition—for example, a bruise to the skin resulting from a blow, or a rash related to measles—refers to common nonspecific reaction as stress. There are certain responses to stress, he notes, that continue in the body much longer than the emergency reactions to the initial "challenge." The responses to stress which occur all over the body serve he believes, to marshall the body's defenses and to protect it from damage.

Since the body's reaction to stress mobilizes the defenses and reduces damage, the response is a beneficial one, and essential for man's survival. This, incidentally, is the approach of much of the physician's efforts in treating a patient to remove interference so that the natural body defenses can most fully contribute to remediation. Generally the response to stress increases the level of resistance to the factor that provoked it, and to similar agents.

However, if stress persists over an extended period of time, the mechanism can cease to function effectively. When this happens, the patient succumbs to the pressures of his illness. At times his resistance to the original resistance is increased, but may decline in regard to other types of stresses.

Reactions to Stress

Almost Anything Can Be Stressful

As has been noted, anything can become stressful if it is "strong enough, lasts long enough, or is repeated often enough." Since our minds are involved in everything that happens to us, the *anything*, as we have observed, may be physical or emotional, with almost any emotionally upsetting condition—fear or anxiety—triggering off the stress response and the physical reaction associated with it. The upsets, as we have observed are at times fairly easy to identify: severe illness, the death of a loved one, a fight, anticipated surgery, loss of a job, or another serious problem. Stress can also be activated by less obvious factors: an examination, a fear of rejection or domination, or almost any other challenging or threatening situation with which a person may be confronted.

Usually the stress sets off so mild a reaction as to operate without the immediate knowledge of the participant. Only later does the person recall that his heart was beating faster, that he was perspiring more heavily than usual, or that his breathing was more labored.

As we have pointed out, the mere expectation of a stressful event, uncertainty, or strangeness can often be as stressful as the event itself. Also, new or confounding occurrences may trigger stress.

Coping

Sometimes, when one realizes that a particular situation is not dangerous, the stress reaction, though initiated, shuts itself off. Often even if one cannot figure out the situation entirely but has an idea of how to handle it, the reaction can also be shut off.

We have observed, too, that a brief, successful bout with stress can usually help to strengthen resistance by enhancing the body's capacity to overcome it and similar pressures without developing a stress reaction. In other words, by learning to master pressures, we can help to control and reduce future bouts which would normally induce stress.[39] Most people have learned how to cope with basic, every-day life occurrences. They have learned how to relate to others, how to defer unpleasant tasks, how to try to forget their problems.

But no one is entirely invulnerable.

When there is constant pressure upon us, or when things get more difficult than we expect, or when we are not too sure how things will work out, we begin to worry, which can trigger the stress response.

If the body has a weakened, damaged, or vulnerable part, severe stress, particularly of a long-term chronic nature, may cause serious physical damage. Most people seem to have an inherent physiological weakness somewhere, so that while one person may respond to continuing stress by developing an ulcer, another might have a heart attack, and a third, an asthma attack.

Association of Thoughts With Previous Attacks

Harris spells out even further the close interplay between emotional and physical factors.[40] He describes the interaction between the two as a "Pavlovian-like" conditioned reflex, which associates stressful thoughts and experiences with previous attacks. The emotions prepare the autonomic nervous system, so that excitants which at one time could not provoke reactions, become able to do so. The "associative factors" would appear to facilitate the repetition of attacks by linking together the memory of an attack with the particular stressors.

Enter the Allergen

Harris also suggests the possibility that impulses, emotional in nature, "that emanate from the higher brain centers" can increase the permeability of the blood vessel barrier, with the individual becoming more susceptible to infection and allergy.

When this occurs, allergens penetrate the vessels, the blood supply is augmented to some susceptible organ or tissue, thereby promoting the union of antigen and antibody.

The process is seen most clearly in disorders which are labeled "psychogenic," where the role of the emotional factors in the development of physical illness is more easily discernible. The process may more clearly be seen in the several illustrations which follow.

Psychogenic Disorders

Emotional Factors in the Development of Coronary Attacks

An addition to the growing literature of the interplay of mind and body, is a study on the role of personality and emotion in heart-attack patients conducted by Drs. Meyer Friedman and Roy Rosenman of Mt. Zion Hospital's Harold Brunn Institute.[41] In extensive studies lasting eight and a half years, the researchers determined that "personality types" were a significant factor in heart attacks, and were even more important than obesity, high blood pressure, or smoking. They observed that 90 percent of patients under the age of 60 who had heart attacks, had "unique" personality traits.

On the basis of psychosocial data obtained during interviews, the doctors divided their patients into high-risk and low-risk groups. The high-risk group (Type A) had twice as many heart attacks as the low risk (Type B). The researchers found that type A's coronaries were also twice as likely to be fatal as type B's and that A's who survived their first coronary, had a much greater chance of suffering a second attack than type B's.

Who Were the Type A's? The doctors observed a number of common emotional characteristics in the type A's. These people seemed to be living under almost "unbearable stress." They appeared to have set up for themselves "impossible expectations," and their life style was characterized as a "chronic and continuous struggle."

Some of the outward expressions of the inner turmoil which the doctors observed in these people were:

—they were habitually impatient;

—they were in a state of almost constant stress, with an urgent feeling that they never had "enough time";

—their speech was hurried and explosive;

—their bodies constantly appeared tense, and never relaxed;

—their body movements were brisk;

—they were often obsessed with numbers—with the amount of sales made, articles written, forms completed;

—they were prone to vent their hostility in verbal abuse, even on family and friends.

Who Were the Type B's? By contrast, the type B's didn't seem to be as emotionally charged as the A's. They did not rush to judgments, or make snap decisions, and they refrained from antagonizing even their subordinates.

Together with the personality differences, the doctors observed a correlation of important physical symptoms which they believe result from type A's stress: these included higher cholesterol, increased norepinepherine, increased ACTH (a hormone that stimulates the adrenal glands), and low levels of growth hormone.

Though other psychological, social, and environmental factors related to heart attack no doubt exist in addition to the biological and physical features noted in the study, the statistical and biochemical evidence from Mount Zion seems to point clearly to the important relationship of emotion and life style to heart disease—so much so that in the opinion of the principal researchers, if the A personality type is not modified, and if his perpetual struggle is not abated, he will remain a prime heart attack prospect, and regardless of changes which he may introduce in his diet, exercise, or in his smoking habits, "unless his personality is modified, these will do but little good."

Emotion And Rheumatoid Arthritis

Another account which similarly points to the very close relationship between emotional factors and organic illness is offered by Dr. Alan J. Rose of the Department of Physical Medicine at Addenbrooks Hospital in Cambridge, England.[42] In a *Medical World News* report, Dr. Rose suggests that dramatic improvement in cases of rheumatoid arthritis could frequently be achieved by the treatment of emotional difficulties.

Dr. Rose attempts first to draw some distinction between what he calls "psychosomatic rheumatism," where symptoms are expressions of anxiety, tension, or depressive illness, and "true" rheumatoid arthritis, though he sees both as serious, painful, and real. He believes however, that in the former, the treatment of the underlying psychopathology usually results in fairly rapid improvement in symptoms. Dr. Rose observes, that even the true rheumatoid has an emotional overtone, and even if significant improvement is not achieved in the condition itself by psychological means, "a dramatic improvement in responses to anti-rheumatic drugs may occur if the underlying depression is also vigorously treated." In other words an emotional component appears to be present in both rheumatisms. In the former, alleviation appears to bring on dramatic improvement; in the latter, when conflicts have been resolved, responsiveness to medication appears to be better.

Emotion And Duodonal Ulcers

A third illustration relates to the work of Dr. H. Weiner on duodonal ulcers in 2,000 army recruits.[43] This study perhaps illustrates even more clearly the thesis that we have been attempting to develop.

After comprehensive testing of the soldiers—including physical, emotional, and sociological factors—Weiner, in describing what seems to have occurred, perceived of the reaction which precipitated their ulcers as taking place on three tiers or layers. The first, he determined, occurred on a physiological tier. This was characterized by an elevated level of "serum pep-

sinogen" in their system. Second, he observed a unique profile—a "susceptible personality" (to ulcer)—and third, he noticed unique "external life circumstances" as contributing or
precipitating factors in their illness.

Instruction For Asthma

Dr. Pinkerton sees a very close similarity between the three
tiers which precipitate duodonal ulcers and those in the asthmatic individual.[44] The first (1) is vulnerability to allergens,
which (2) primes an unstable, or "labile" bronchus. The third
(3) is "external life circumstances" which may precipitate an
attack. According to this theory, for asthma to occur there
must be physical predisposition interacting with a psychological predisposition (a susceptible personality). The attack ultimately occurs or is triggered by emotional or stressful factors.

What we seem to have here are complex factors contributing to, and precipitating illness: rheumatoid arthritis, coronary attacks, ulcers, and asthma. We are presented in effect
with a multicausal theory of illness from which we can see
asthma arising from intertwining influences. In the latter case
(asthma), these influences include physical vulnerability,
which results from predisposed physical and hereditary influences; susceptibility to offending allergens; and stress imposed
by the social and psychological setting.

The asthma-causing culprit may then be a single factor, but
more probably a number of factors—immunological and physical—acting in concert; possibly a labile bronchus; offending allergens such as foods, dust, mites, or pollen; infections, tension,
and fatigue; and adverse life circumstances, which may include emotional factors such as excitement, frustration, anger,
fear, or other forms of social stress.

Vulnerability. That vulnerability, or "genetic predisposition,"
is fundamental to the condition, is seen even by Dr. M. Murray Peshkin, the dean of American allergists who is generally
prone to place emphasis on the emotional components of
asthma. Dr. Peshkin cautions that we should not be led to believe that the illness can be induced "in any person who is not

genetically predisposed to asthma," and stresses that environmental tensions seem to be the secondary contributing factor. Though emotions are apparently a significant contributing factor to the illness, we must bear in mind that they are certainly not the exclusive cause.

The Labile Bronchus. Bruce Pearson has identified an important physical feature in asthmatics which he calls the "labile bronchus."[45] Since it is the bronchial tract which is principally involved in the illness, he sees the ready capability of the bronchus for change as a primary problem. The labile or unstable bronchus, according to Pearson, contracts excessively at a variety of stimuli which include chemical, physical, or biological changes. Similarly, the bronchus at times overreacts to inhaled isoprenaline.

Some have attempted to classify asthma by type: allergic, infective, and psychogenic. It appears, as Peshkin has indicated, that all asthma has an immunological basis, irrespective of infections and allergens, but that many cases may be affected by emotions.

Dr. Philip Pinkerton of the University of Liverpool feels that "all three (allergic, infective and psychogenic) contributions obtain but that they are complimentary in action, not mutually exclusive, so that their clinical impact is summative [the total effect of the various components] and not disparate [individual]."

Mind and Body

Unity of The Body and Mind

The eminent psychiatrist Dr. John Schwab reminds us that the theory of "unity of the body and the mind," and "multiple causation," which is making a comeback today, were understood and practiced for hundreds of years by the physicians of antiquity, but later fell into disuse.[46] "Our present emphasis on comprehensive medical care," he writes, "is a return to

concepts once accepted as indisputable—the essential unity of
the mind and body, a basic tenet of Greco-Roman medicine,
which was artificially divided by Christian theology."

Unity of the Organism and the Environment

The noted social scientist Dr. Kurt Lewin provides us in his
famed "field theory" with an integrated understanding of the
comprehensive nature of illness which goes beyond a mere
need to understand body and mind.[47] To Lewin, the field is
"the totality of co-existing facts which are mutually inter-
dependent." He sees a constant and ongoing interdependence
of the organism and the environment, with the two never
existing in isolation of each other, but constantly interacting
and influencing one another.

As such, to Lewin and to many others there are no purely
"psychosomatic diseases." A relationship exists between physical and mental illness and social factors. The consequence of
all illness is to an extent influenced by the social environment.

Since the person is so complex, an understanding of his illness requires a thorough knowledge of him in his totality
Schwab goes so far as to say that to evaluate each patient effectively, the physician must employ the "tools of anthro-
pology, sociology, and psychology."[48]

But most doctors cannot operate this way. Physicians, as a
result of their training, seek in the main to isolate single
causes for illness. They are encouraged in their search for the
identification of specific factors leading to an illness, so that
when they have discovered or isolated the "particular" cause,
they may proceed to prescribe a specific remedy. In the process, they often overlook the effect of the patient's state of
mind, and of emotional and environmental factors on his
health.

As far back as the fifth century B.C., Hippocrates, the philosopher-physician observed that to be successful, it was necessary for doctors to "have knowledge of the whole of things"—
to see the entire patient, to understand in as comprehensive a
manner as possible just what makes him tick. The famed He-

brew philosopher-physician Maimonides, in his study of
asthma written nearly eight hundred years ago, stressed that
the physician must treat the patient, not merely the illness.
When the physician diagnoses, he writes, "he must see the patient and his illness in context, and when he prescribes, he
must seek a remedy for the total patient, not merely for the
illness which can never really be separated from the total person."[49]

Treating the Whole Person

There is a need then to treat the whole person, not just the
disease. In 1898 Sir William Osler observed, "A good physician treats the disease, a *great* physician treats the patient."[50]
Since few physicians have the time to be "great," there is need
for the effort of a team—physician, allergist, dietician—to afford the basic medical treatment, to desensitize the patient
against offending allergens, to prescribe effective anti-
spasmodic medication, to suggest a suitable diet, and for a behavioral therapist to become involved in the emotional area.

5

PARENTECTOMY AND INSTITUTIONALIZATION

Peshkin's Theory

Dr. Murray Peshkin was the first to employ the term "parentectomy" to describe a condition which he observed over 50 years ago at New York's Mount Sinai Hospital.[51] While serving in the hospital's pediatric ward with the noted physician Bela Schick, Dr. Peshkin noted that a goodly number of children brought in for treatment for severe asthma showed remarkable improvement within hours or days after arriving at the hospital. The remissions, he observed, frequently came about "without the use of medications or special treatment."

Searching for the reason for the improvement, Dr. Peshkin speculated that it might be the antiseptic atmosphere of the hospital. The doctor relates that investigation proved to him, though, that the amount of pollutants and allergens present at the hospital, which bounds Fifth Avenue, with its heavy traffic and exhaust fumes, and Central Park, with its abundance of trees, grass, and dust, could hardly be considered an improved atmosphere over the homes of many of the young patients. He observed, "Since some of the children came from homes which were only one hundred feet away from the hospital, and others lived within a few miles of the hospital, I knew that within these geographic limits there was no climatic condition which could account for the observed results."

In a paper published in 1930 in the *American Journal of Disease of Children*, Dr. Peshkin indicated that the physical relocation of the homes of asthmatic children and removal of furniture proved ineffective in providing relief for the bulk of the youngsters whom he had seen.

He writes:

Moving the home from one section of the city to another proved an economic hardship and a costly failure. The removal of furniture, draperies, carpets, articles of apparel and other substances, as well as carriers known to cause allergy (until in some cases the interior of the home took on the appearance of an army barracks) proved of no avail.

The floors and the walls were scrubbed with various dilutions of mercuric chloride. The solution was kept in contact with the surface to which it was applied for at least one half hour, but this proved ineffective ... I originally believed that perhaps the physical removal of the child with intractable asthma from a hyper-allergenic home environment to a hypo-allergenic hospital environment, accounted for the benefits which we experienced in the hospital. As a result, I saw to it that the most scrupulous attempts were made to render the child's home environment as hypoallergenic as possible ... [including removal of] all objects which might have been the source of allergens to which the child might have been hypersensitive. Despite all these precautions, including what is considered to constitute adequate hyposensitivity therapy, the child who had been free of his allergenic bronchial asthma in the hospital, nearly always developed asthma the night of his homecoming—or at the very latest within several days of his release from the hospital.

... On the other hand, the removal of the child usually in a condition of "status asthmaticus" to the ward of the hospital, resulted in the majority of instances in complete relief of all symptoms of asthma within the first three days after admission, and freedom from asthma was maintained during the entire stay in the hospital. *However, when the child was returned to its home, asthma recurred within several days, and most often on the first night.* [italics mine][52]

Puzzled by these strange occurrences, Peshkin sought to understand the reason for the remission from status asthma in a large number of cases upon admission to the hospital, and for the recurrence of the condition upon their return home.

Following extensive observation, he concluded that the major factor which had changed upon their admission to the hospital, was the youngsters' separation from their parents. He thus coined the term "parentectomy" to describe the separation and ensuing remission.

Peshkin's Theory Tested

Peshkin was able to test his theory later over a period of several decades while he served as director of the Children's Asthmatic Research Institute and Hospital (CARIH) in Denver.

Studying thousands of youngsters who came to his facility for treatment, he observed that the Denver altitude and atmospheric conditions did not always represent an improvement over those cities, towns, and villages from which the young patients came.

He noted parenthetically, "The Denver situation is not very much different than the experience at Mt. Sinai. Even though Denver is a mile high, the pollen and mold concentration nearly always exceeds many areas of the country from which the children originally came."[53]

Nevertheless, a significant number showed dramatic improvement in their asthma, merely upon admittance to the facility, when they were separated from their families. Peshkin thus felt that his theory of "parentectomy" was reconfirmed.

Visiting Day Attacks

Peshkin also paid close attention to the reaction of the children on visiting days. He writes:

When I repeatedly observed a child in a convalescent home rendered symptom-free by his separation from his home environment, and that a visit by his mother could precipitate a major attack of asthma, I realized then, more than ever, that hospitalization and the removal of a child to a convalescent home, was in effect the separation of the child from the asthmatogenic emotional climate which existed in the child's own home, and that it was this adverse psychogenic factor which was principally responsible for sending the asthmatic child into a state of intractable asthma.[54,55]

Support For Peshkin's Theory

Peshkin's observations about the role of parents in the illness appear to have support from numerous researchers. In 1958, Long sought to determine whether the creation of antiseptic conditions for asthmatics really mattered as much as an improved psychological climate.[56] Convinced that there were factors other than purely medical ones operating within the institutional setting which contributed to the improved condition of asthma patients, Long set out to explore whether the improvement of highly allergic children within the hospital was actually due to their isolation from allergenic substances. In an innovative experiment, he had his assistants collect the contents of vacuum cleaner bags which contained the actual dust from the homes of a number of patients at an asthma hospital. He then introduced the dust from their own homes into the ventilation ducts which led to the patients' rooms at the hospital. Interestingly, the young patients whose medical records in the main indicated "dust sensitive," remained virtually unaffected by the presence of this normally highly allergenic substance in their atmosphere.

Experiment With Substitute Parents

If Peshkin's observation had laid the groundwork for the concept of "parentectomy," and Long had proved that separation from home allergens was not a vital factor in remission, investigation by psychologist, Ken Purcell, illustrated even more dramatically that it was rarely the physical setting from which the institutionalized child came, nor the atmosphere or contents of a particular home, that influenced his condition, but that it was rather the emotional quality of the setting, and the child's interaction with the people within the setting, which were most important.[57]

Purcell arranged for professional housemothers to assume normal child-rearing responsibilities within the actual home of asthmatic youths for a two-week period, while the children's biological parents were provided with a paid vacation away from both their children and home. Brothers and sisters went on vacation with their parents, while the asthmatic children remained at home with their substitute mothers. During the period of the families' absence, a significant reduction in the frequency of asthmatic attacks was noted, as was a reduction in the amount of medication required. This study appears to be particularly revealing since the actual homes of the children were utilized, and exposure to physical factors and allergens within or about the residences remained precisely the same as that which existed when the family was present.

Though there is need for additional study in the entire area of "parentectomy," one thing is fairly certain—that the concept of "surrogate parents"—professional housemothers moving into a child's home—and parents and siblings exiting, is neither a desired nor a realistic arrangement for most families of asthmatic children.

Institutionalization

Advantages of Institutionalization

Is institutionalization, then, a suitable alternative? Several of the asthmatic children's facilities have claimed dramatic improvement rates for patients, a prominent one recently reported a remission rate of over 80 percent.

Apparently there is significant benefit in custodial care for many youngsters. The institutional setting would appear to be particularly useful to the child who cannot because of difficult home conditions have his basic needs attended to. It may merit serious consideration, too, for the family which is not physically capable of providing for its child or for the intractably ill or debilitated child for whom treatment alternatives are lacking. It might also be useful for a child whose health is aggravated by a charged psychological climate at home, or for the child from a parentless home, or from a one-parent home with a working mother or father, or where other factors prevent the child from satisfying his basic physical, social, and emotional needs.

Disagreement Over Institutional Claims

It should be noted that some fundamental conflict exists among leading allergists in regard to the degree of remission achieved within the institutional setting for the bulk of patients. Dr. Constantine J. Falliers, reporting on a fifteen-year study of the treatment of asthmatic children in a residential center, found a significant reduction in the number of remissions reported from the earlier to the later years of the study. Figures for the earlier dates reported a remission rate of 98 percent (only 2 percent showed no improvement in the institution). By the middle of the study only 38 percent showed significant improvement, and by the end of the study the figure had fallen to 12 percent. Whether these reduced improvement figures represent a change in the method of record keeping, or whether the availability of remedial medications during the latter phases on the outside had begun to leave just a "hard core" of patients for the institutions, is open to speculation. Dr. Falliers points out that despite a "controlled environment" in the institution, and constant medical supervision of all the children, "episodes of status asthmaticus are not rare." As such the doctor concludes that they [the residential treatment facilities] "should not be expected to offer miraculous cures, when in most instances the therapeutic team in the patient's own community, aided by modern specialized techniques, can offer adequate clinical services much sooner, more consistently, and for a longer period of time."[58]

Since criteria for admission to a residential facility for the asthmatic child lack specificity, and the criteria for sending them home are likewise open to question, a number of basic questions remain to be answered: When should a child be discharged? When his symptoms disappear? When his condition is stabilized? When there is a reduction in the number of attacks? When the child has displayed an improved ability to function with others?

Since institutionalization of the asthmatic youngster is at times necessary, its long-term benefits to both the patient and his family should be examined. Are the positive results achieved in the institution offset upon his return home? The extent to which the benefits are lasting when an "improved child" returns to the environment which may have contributed to, precipitated, or aggravated his condition initially, has not really been studied adequately.

How real is the institutional setting, with its reduced emotional stress, constant doctoring, and controlled environment? It may well be that the most beneficial effect of the process is for the parents, who "meanwhile get a wholesome recess from the emotions, financial, and social pressures of having a chronically ill child at home."

It is instructive to attend staff conferences at a number of residential institutions before the major holidays and observe the deliberations and apprehensions of staff in regard to allowing "improved" children to go home for a few days. Peshkin's comment that "the flare-up of the asthma often occurred within hours after the child returned home," is often very much on the mind of staff charged with the responsibility of arranging the child's return to his home.[59] Behaviorists and allergists have seen a child's condition aggravated following a visit to the hospital or institution by family members, and even more evidence of relapse when the child returns to unimproved psychological home conditions for a holiday or summer vacation.

Institutionalization, then, which often lasts from eighteen months to two years, is recommended only when home conditions are difficult and when other methods of treatment have failed or do not portend to be beneficial—in short, only in selective cases.

Residential Costs and Capacity

It must be noted too that the capacity of residential facilities is exceedingly limited; the total bed capacity in the nation for chronic asthmatic children requiring long-term residential treatment is approximately 600, and the cost is
prohibitively high for the average family. The expense, for example, of providing lodging, schooling, medical, and psychological care, and the other needs of a youthful patient at the
Children's Asthmatic Research Institute and Hospital in Denver, at the time of this writing is in excess of $20,000 annually
and is rapidly increasing.

Again, the concern more overriding than the availability of
space and high cost, and which should be carefully weighed
by the family considering institutionalization, is what happens
to the child discharged from the institution after spending a
year or more there? Many allergists and behaviorists feel that
the chances for recurrence of the former asthmatic condition
are high unless some significant change has occurred within
the family while the child has been away.

A Need for Change in the Family

Sperling questions the long-term improvement potential and
the intrinsic value of institutionalization unless the parents are
involved in the "change process." He notes that asthmatic
children

respond to environmental manipulation, but the asthmatic core remains, with crippling effects to the child. We know of the beneficial
results of hospitalization and residential treatment . . . but these
methods of dealing with the child's illness are of limited value because they do not effect basic changes in the personality of the
child . . . *unless the child is treated, and in many cases, particularly of young
children, unless the parents are also treated, no lasting results will be achieved.*
[italics mine][60]

It stands to reason that the return of the "cured" patient to
the setting from which he previously came, barring change on

the families' part, is almost analagous to returning a juvenile delinquent fresh out of "correctional school" to his former neighborhood, with all of the attendant social and environmental factors which no doubt contributed to his delinquent behavior in the first place.

Health Village

Perhaps asthma sufferers and their families may some day benefit from the "health village" concept, which will be able to combine both physical and emotional care for the entire family. A prototype of such a village, (though not catering to asthmatics) is located in Sweden, at Lake Malar, a short distance from Stockholm. Here 30 families live, half of whom see themselves as having problems, the rest, the staff members who treat them. The village is comprised in the main of insular families who are passive and withdrawn. While the program is voluntary, the parents, according to Dr. Bengt Borjeson, a former dean of the Stockholm University School of Social Work, who runs the therapeutic community, "are compelled by their own unhappiness to seek help." Started as a residential treatment center for children, it was later transformed into a "family center" in the belief "that treating a child alone often ignores the fact that he comes from, and will return to, a disturbed family situation. It also ignores the ability of the family to help itself get better."[61]

Though villages of this type, where the entire family can live, learn, work, and be treated together, may some day become a reality for asthmatics in this country and abroad, for the present they represent an ideal rather than a real situation, and are greatly beyond the reach of the average family. The project and proposal which we discuss later may come a bit closer to fullfilling current needs in a more realistic manner.

6

SUGGESTIBILITY AND THERAPY

Recognition of the relationship between asthma and emotion dates back more than 2,000 years, to the days of Hippocrates, who observed that "If the asthmatic is to master his condition, he must guard against his own anger." Many of the ancient physicians—Galen, Aretaeus, Maimonides, and their successors—similarly identified the connection between asthma and emotion.

In the last century, Trousseau, a French physician who himself suffered from asthma, described in 1858 an asthmatic attack which he had. He related how anger over the discovery of his wagon driver's thievery precipitated a severe attack of asthma from barn dust. He indicated that at other times, when his emotions were not aroused, exposure to the same barn dust did not bring on asthma.

Several years later, in 1886, the physician MacKenzie described how a patient who was known to be allergic to roses, had an acute asthmatic attack upon being exposed to an artificial rose. He observed that the flower had been previously cleaned, so that no dust or irritant could possibly have been on it.

Psychological Influence

To what extent do psychological factors or suggestion influence asthma attacks?

Dr. Thomas Luparello, head of the Department of Behavioral Research at the National Jewish Hospital and Research Center in Denver, and his associates reported in the *New York State Journal of Medicine* on a unique experiment that they had conducted.[62]

A group of 40 asthmatic patients were informed that they were part of a study related to the control of air pollution, and that the researchers were trying to determine the concentration of substances in the atmosphere which would induce attacks of wheezing. Each patient was told that he would be inhaling five different concentrations of an irritant or allergen which had previously been associated with his asthma attacks. The patients were led to believe that they would be exposed to increasing amounts of the irritants or allergens when in reality they were inhaling plain saline solutions.

Nineteen of the 40 patients reacted with significant airway obstruction. Twelve of these 19 went on to develop full-blown asthma attacks, including wheezing and dyspnea (shortness of breath).

At a later date, 29 of the original patients were recalled. Fourteen of these had not reacted with significant change after inhaling the substance, while 15 had. Of the 15 reactors in the first study, all 15 reacted again. Fourteen of the 29 patients who had not reacted the first time, remained nonreactive.

Of particular interest was another aspect of the study, in which there was a reduction of asthma symptoms, with attacks clearing in all instances—as patients were told that allergens and other irritants were being withdrawn from their inhalants, and that isoproterenol hydrochloride was being introduced—when in effect only placebos (inert replacements) were being used throughout the experiment.

In addition to highlighting the suggestibility inherent in a significant number of cases of asthma, the researchers' latter finding may be significant in evaluating the effectiveness of certain medications used in treatment. When improvement occurs, is it due entirely to the pharmacological action of a particular drug? A basic question for us to consider is, to what degree does the expectation of recovery actually enable the patient to improve? Tuft, in a study of 500 asthmatics at the Children's Asthma Research Institute in Denver, Colorado, and Lask, in a detailed study of 100 cases in general practice, support the conclusion that among all the potential influences affecting the asthmatic state, *emotional factors seem to be the most significant.*[63]

Asthmatic Types

Luparello's "highly suggested" patient category (those whose airways became obstructed) comprises somewhat less than half (47.5 percent) of the total number of asthmatics whom he studied. It is interesting that Ken Purcell observed that a slightly lower figure, about 40 percent of juvenile patients admitted to a leading asthma residential facility, "rapidly remitted" from their symptoms shortly after their admission. This group remained virtually symptom-free and required almost no medication. The others who did not rapidly remit, he observed, were higher in steroid dependencies, and required continuous dosages of cortisone drugs.

In extensive studies comparing characteristics of the rapidly remitting to the steroid-dependent children, Purcell noted that emotional factors "anger, anxiety, and depression" appeared to be involved significantly in the triggering of asthmatic attacks of the former. In-depth study of the parents of the rapidly remitting children showed them to be much more authoritative and punitive than the parents of the others. Purcell concluded that the illness of this group may be associated with "neurotic conflicts" and "affective reactions" to a much greater extent than that of the others.

A Comparison Between Rapidly Remitting and Steroid-Dependent Children

Purcell's study points to a significantly high percentage of youngsters in the "rapidly remitting" group from psychologi-

cally "unhealthy" settings. Not only did the youngsters display
more neurotic symptoms but they appeared to be from more
disturbed backgrounds. There was a higher incidence of au-
thoritarian control in their families, and a significantly higher
amount of hostility and rejection of the youngsters by the
mothers.

Although there were many noteworthy personality distur-
bances in the steroid-dependent youngsters as well, and much
research into the psychological and pathological role of
asthma in their condition remains to be done, Purcell's study
suggests that the asthmatic syndrome might be "more likely to
be acquired as a mode of response to coping with psychological stress or conflict."[64] The hypothesis follows that "the removal of these children from a stressful interpersonal environment would reduce the necessity for using the asthmatic
syndrome." Simply stated, this study appears to confirm Peshkin's observations of parentectomy and other environmental
factors at work, and suggests that asthma could conceivably be
controlled in approximately 40 percent of cases if the stressful
environment could be modified or eliminated.

Changing the Environment

The residential setting discussed in the previous chapter, as
unrealistic as it might be, may in this regard incorporate supportive features, not only because it separates children from
their parents but equally because of its protective environment, in which the child feels accepted, and in which he sees
himself as not being too different from those about him. Since
the bulk of the population has similar physical characteristics,
the child does not stand out by virtue of his illness. He is
among his own, and can function in what to him is a more
normal environment.

Grouping asthmatic youngsters with other asthmatics may
in itself have therapeutic value. The Swedish pediatric physician Krakelien sees meaningful benefits in such groupings.
"For psychological reasons," he writes, "it is important that
chronically sick children should not feel that their difference
makes them inferior." Krakelien sees this as a value of the

residential treatment facility. "In a special asthmatic convalescent home where the child is not an exception," he continues, "their physical handicaps do not seem to be such a
drawback . . ."[65]

Alternatives to Institutionalization

Since it is highly unlikely that we will ever be able to remove our reported asthma population of 8 or 9 million from
their stressful environment to group residential settings, alternate ways of enabling them to cope must be explored.

The most sensible appears to be to keep them at home and
to attempt to identify and work through anxieties, stress, fears,
and assorted tensions which seem to contribute to their condition.

Individual or Family Therapy

A number of alternate methods to help the patient and his
family understand and work on feelings and responses to given
stimuli are possible. To effectively achieve this goal, an intensive program of individual, or preferably family therapy would
be indicated. If skillfully administered, such a regimen could
succeed in opening vistas of understanding, and an appreciation of the dynamics of interaction within the family constellation. The parents' feelings for each other, their attitude
toward the asthmatic child and toward the other children,
could thus be studied and understood. But the process of family or individual therapy can be a lengthy and costly one.

The Group Program

A viable and perhaps even more effective alternative is rehabilitation through the small social group.

The small social or therapy group is a quasi-family situation
in which the individual is constantly relating to others, acting
out, and testing his conflicts and emotions. When the others in

the group are asthmatics, there is not only shared common interest but, as Krakelien has pointed out, a *shared disability* which encourages support and self-expression by reducing the feeling of isolation that the chronically ill youngster often experiences on the "outside."

There is provision within the group for reality testing. The group presents the individual with a chance to compare himself to others like him and to notice how they respond, acclimate, and adjust to each other and to their illness.

Theodore H. Wohl, too, sees the group as the "natural setting for [the individual] to work through his conflicts." He observes that the "individual is above all a social being, a product of intrapsychic forces, as well as of biological drives." and suggests that "the group would appear to be a natural setting for experiencing and working through interpersonal, as well as intrapersonal conflicts."[66]

The advantages of the group setting, Wohl feels, is that it offers an opportunity of relating not only to individuals, but to a miniature community as well. He notes "Within the group, the person is able to communicate on a one to one basis." As a group member, he may experience his nuclear family constellation.

Value of the Group. What can the social or therapy group achieve? Its primary goals are to socialize and rehabilitate. In addition to working toward improved physical functioning, the groups strive to enhance the social functioning of participants, to help in their growth needs, in the development of social responsibilities, and in improved interpersonal relations.

Through the media of dynamics and programming, the group can provide experiences to help the individual grow both emotionally and socially. For the physically or emotionally handicapped person the group can also focus naturally on remedial goals: restoration and rehabilitation. It helps prevent social breakdown, and provides corrective experiences in those instances where individual or social breakdown has occurred.

The group leader or therapist likewise has the advantage of seeing the patient relating to individuals and to the group family. The therapist can help him to utilize either or both experiences for his benefit. "As the individual communicates in the group," Wohl notes, "an observant therapist may notice his pattern of behavior to others and how he is influenced by various stimuli provided by the group.[67]

Groups for Parents

The group offers an excellent therapeutic setting not only for the asthmatic child, but for his parents as well.

Dr. Joseph E. Ghory of the Convalescent Hospital for Children at the University of Cincinnatti Medical School, is a firm believer in the value of parents' groups. "We have placed much less emphasis on psychotherapy for the child," he reports,

and much more emphasis on psychotherapy for the parents. To this end we have instituted group psychotherapy sessions for the mothers of asthmatic children . . . more recently we have inaugurated similar group psychotherapy sessions for the fathers as well. In addition to the prime value of educating the parents to the disease itself, the group sessions have allowed the parents to ventilate their feelings of anxiety, apprehension, and concern over their children, and when it exists, their own frustrated feelings of anger and hostility.[68]

The ideal situation would appear to be separate therapy groups for both children and parents.

In the next chapter we describe the development and functioning of a number of experimental small social therapy groups operating separately for asthmatic children and their parents, and evaluate their effectiveness in the reduction of asthma symptomology.

7

THE HADASSA EXPERIMENT

Hadassa, Tel Aviv's oldest hospital, is one of three health facilities comprising the government municipal hospital system of Tel Aviv. Located in the heart of Israel's bustling metropolis, the hospital serves the city's resident population of 650,000, which increases to nearly a million in the day time, when suburban commuters are drawn to the city's factories, shopping facilities, and beaches.

The hospital is housed in a series of buildings located just a stone's throw from Allenby Road, which is the main artery carrying traffic from the heart of industrial Tel Aviv to its glistening Mediterranean beaches. As Allenby Road approaches the hospital, it touches the border of the teeming pushcart-filled Carmel Market, the largest fruit, vegetable, and sundry open-air shopping market in the city, and probably in all of Israel. The road then continues along the outskirts of the bustling, picturesque Yemenite Quarter, with its narrow cobblestone streets, crowded buildings, and huddled population existing amid a multitude of Oriental food stores, cafés, and outdoor restaurants, from which there constantly emanates the fragrance of charcoal-broiled meats and other exotic eastern aromas. Allenby Road ends about half a mile past Hadassa at Israel's Riviera, the beachfront which contains the ultramodern hotels which house a large number of Israel's tourists.

Situated as it is in the midst of a diversified population, the hospital may at almost any time count among its patients a cross-section of Tel Aviv's citizenry—poor and middle-class men and women, working people who have been brought to the hospital for emergency treatment of factory accidents, and a sprinkling of wealthy tourists in need of medical attention, for whom Hadassa is the most accessible hospital.

Hadassa, a general hospital with the wide range of services associated with a large city hospital, also contains a number of out-patient departments. Among them is an allergy clinic. Israel's largest facility of this type.

The Project

Incidence of Asthma in Tel Aviv

A recent Israel Ministry of Health survey indicated that 21 out of 1,000 school-age children in the city, that is, 2.1 percent, are asthmatics. Since school age in Israel, means roughly ages 5 to 14, it would appear that the figure for the total youth population, aged 1 to 16, exceeds 2.1 percent, and would probably be comparable to the estimated 3 percent of the American youth population who are believed to be afflicted with an asthma-related illness.[69]

Participants in the Project

The Hadassa Allergy Clinic served as the setting for an exciting research experiment into the possibility of rehabilitating asthmatic youngsters through the medium of small social therapy groups. The project developed by the author in association with the School of Social Work of the Bar Ilan University in Ramat Gan (a Tel Aviv suburb) consisted of five therapy groups for asthmatic youngsters aged 6 to 13. Each group was comprised of 6 to 7 children of similar age and the same sex. Corresponding groups for mothers of these children were also established.

The children selected for the project had serious chronic bronchial asthma which was intractable, i.e., their condition was unresponsive to treatment, and was leading to a gradual decrease in their vital lung capacity.

The Intake Session

An intensive psychosocial intake interview was arranged for each youngster and mother to determine a variety of socialization factors. Included were evaluations of how the patient viewed himself and his family, feelings about home conditions, how he related to his brothers, sisters, and friends, and how he felt about his illness.

An attempt was made during intake to receive from mothers an overview of the child's social and medical history—to hear of any problems which they believed they or their child was facing as a result of his illness, and to discuss specific concerns regarding the child's ability to relate to friends and siblings.

This session also served as an opportunity to inform both mothers and children separately about the program, the group, the leaders, and the methods that would be used at upcoming sessions.

A comprehensive medical examination including a chest x-ray and blood and urine analysis was arranged to ascertain that each child in the program was infection-free. Pulmonary capacity was measured by a respirometer to determine the amount of air each child was capable of expiring from his lungs in a given, limited time.

The Spirometric Test

Testing the expiratory volume of an individual against a capacity which is considered normal for his age, size, and sex serves as an important barometer in ascertaining the degree of incapacitation from normal respiration. For example, a reduction of a given amount of cubic centimeters from the expected average for a particular age would indicate that a patient's lung capacity has been reduced by a corresponding percentage. Reduced capacity with no significant response following administration of epinepherine implies more limited pulmonary functioning, a reduction in the amount the child is able to expire, and hence a comparable limitation in inspirational (breathing-in) ability, with the attendant implications. Likewise a steady increase in spirometric reading generally points to improved breathing, and shows return to more normal pulmonary capacity and function.

Information Charts

Each mother was given a check list on which to record the frequency and severity of her child's asthma, and to identify sputum, coughing, wheezing, and attacks, as well as amounts of medications used, and other physical and medical phenomena. Like the spirometry tests, these charts were to prove useful in monitoring and in measuring patient progress.

Group Supervision

The children's and mother's groups met separately each week, and were under the leadership of senior social work students of the Bar Ilan University. The students' work was overseen by a university-appointed field supervisor, the director of the Allergy Clinic, and by the Hospital's chief psychiatrist, who met with the students weekly.

Apprehensions

There was understandable apprehension displayed by the children at the outset; they wondered: What are the other children like? What is the group leader like? What does he or she think of me? Will I have to talk about my illness? What is the nature of the activities which we will be participating in? Will I be able to achieve as well as the others?

An effort was made to reduce somewhat the initial anxiety about participating in a hospital-based program by trying to anticipate some of the youngsters' and parents' questions about the nature of the group, and to try to comment on these during the psychosocial interview. For example, the children in the group were to be known as members, not patients; the group was to be known as a club, an "allergy club."

The Children's Groups

The Children's Allergy Club focused on the development of an activity program which sought to gain a better understanding of the youngsters' feelings and to help meet their needs and concerns, while striving to enable them to gain security and confidence.

A variety of activities were offered involving discussion, play, crafts, drama, games, trips, and special events. All were low-pressure activities designed to stimulate participation and to afford reasonable assurance of achievement.

Members were encouraged to articulate their feelings, and to help shape a program based upon their interests and capabilities.

As the youngsters became more comfortable in their group setting, and as they gained confidence in their abilities, the program diversified in both substance and complexity to enable them to build upon the security gained from mastering familiar situations and to move on to newer and more difficult areas with a new-found sense of confidence.

Limitations on physical activity were likewise gradually lifted as the children cultivated a feeling that they could successfully master their environment.

The common bond—all were severe asthmatics—helped reduce both anxietites originating around competition with non-asthmatics, and the feeling of being different, which these youngsters had for too long carried with them and which often placed them at a disadvantage in relating to their peers. Yet the program avoided dwelling on the specific asthma features of the child, discussing the illness only when the child felt like talking about it, and in the main attempting to build upon the healthy parts of the youngster's personality.

Themes. During the course of the sessions the child was encouraged to talk about things which he felt were important to him. He was supported in articulating his feelings, made to feel that they were acceptable, and that he could have his own point of view.

A host of subjects were aired: how the youngsters, who were often moody, depressed, and angry without quite knowing why, saw themselves; how their illness tended to restrict their activities—and how it made them feel different from other children their age, who saw them as weak or sick; the negative feelings that many had about themselves; their frequent feelings that they were failures; their frequent fear of trying new things because they were afraid of failing; their fear of attending outings or activities away from home because of the possibility of having an attack in an unfamiliar setting.

The children also spoke of how they got along with their brothers and sisters, how their siblings felt about their being treated differently, at times receiving special privileges and being babied.

They discussed feelings about how their parents, tried to get them to do their bidding, and to otherwise manipulate them.

As the program continued for a number of weeks, it was observed that apprehensions were reduced. Those who had initially found it difficult to open up, and to express themselves, were begining to do so. The withdrawn members began to associate more easily with the others as they gained friendship and acceptance. As this happened, anxieties diminished some-

what, and relations between the children and staff became
more open.

Leaders. The social work group leaders were warm, accepting, and skillfull in utilizing program media to achieve socialization and involvement. Both verbal and nonverbal activities
were employed, which the club members found not only satisfying socially, but fun and rewarding to participate in. (See
Chapter 12 for exercises to strengthen the muscles of respiration to help clear the airways.)

The staff discovered that the youngsters looked forward ea-
gerly to the weekly meetings, which became for many a high-
light of their week. Though many had to travel considerable
distances from remote parts of the city, or from the outlying
countryside, which for a number meant several bus changes,
the youngsters were pleased to gather each week with other
members of their "allergy club" in the small, spartanly fur-
nished rooms adjacent to the hospital clinic. Play equipment
and program materials were in limited supply, and crafts projects were often constructed from available hospital supplies:
tongue depressors, gauze, adhesive tape, washed out x-ray
plates, and the like.

Initially the hospital courtyard served as the play area for
the children's groups, though children were later taken off hospital grounds to visit local parks, the zoo, a movie, a department store, an observatory, and other places of interest.

The Mother's Groups

Meeting concurrently, but in other rooms apart from their
children, were the various mothers' "clubs." In contrast to the
children's groups which combined verbal and nonverbal activities, the mother's groups were essentially discussion oriented,
seeking to achieve a better understanding of their feelings. A
wide range of topics relating to their feelings about their childrens' illness and its control, and in concepts of child-rearing
permeated the meetings.

The mothers shared their apprehensions about their children's health, and explored approaches to such matters as child-rearing, expectation, limits, punishment, and the child's abilities versus the standards set for him.

The mothers' national origins were varied and represented a number of cultural forms. Countries of origin were as diverse as Israel's variegated population, with families in the program hailing from Romania, Poland, Czechoslovakia, Aden, Greece, Iran, Egypt, Morocco, and Tunisia.

The oft-present feeling that if only they could discover the magic elixir, or if they could but find the *super* doctor somewhere, an instant cure could be achieved, was aired and dispelled. Instead the mothers were encouraged to share their feelings of apprehension, and to achieve increased self-awareness. They were helped to better understand themselves, their families, their children, and the interaction of each upon the other. A wide range of topics of mutual interest were discussed: how the child tends to use his illness, the parents' response to an attack, the climate of the home, sibling relationships, the child's friends, interests, feelings about school, response to allergenic substances, and medication.

Parents' Responses and Feelings. The parents of the asthmatic child often live with a double burden: the child's disability, and their own feelings of inadequacy, guilt, and failure, for almost invariably there is a feeling that to a greater or lesser degree they are to blame for the condition.

The physical and emotional burden of having to care for an ill child for hours at a time, without receiving any emotional support, can prove difficult to the parent and debilitating to the child, and contribute to the deterioration of the lives of the family members.

The groups helped the mothers recognize that the illness did not result from a single factor, but from multicausative factors relating to their child's constitutional vulnerability, physical condition, immunological factors, susceptibility to allergens, as well as to his capacity to cope with family trauma and the stressful situations imposed by society.

When the mothers were able to talk out their problems with someone who was available to listen, their anguish in feeling alone and vulnerable was eased. As they examined their child's behavior and their responses to and interaction with him, their fears were somewhat allayed, and their guilt feelings understood. From this often flowed a modification of their attitudes, actions, and behavior toward their child.

Support of the mothers in the groups often saw the defusing of potentially explosive family crises, and a new understanding resulting in the ongoing care of and concern for their child.

The mothers' response to the program was positive: they were being afforded an opportunity to express their feelings and discuss their problems. Though they were not too certain what bearing these discussions had on their children's condition, there was a feeling of relief on their part that something positive was being done for their child. The relief was all the more welcome for the mother who had come to believe that she was responsible for her child's problems, and had been laden with guilt especially when the child took ill—with a condition that neighbors and friends suspected as having "emotional" overtones.

Parental Change. In subsequent stages the mothers' attitudes underwent considerable change. The initial feelings of guilt were followed by relief: since they were beginning to do something tangible for their child, they could not be "all that bad." At this stage there was a mixture of curiosity regarding the approach used, coupled with a good amount of suspicion.

The next stage offered further reinforcement resulting from a recognition from others in the group that they too had similar problems. At about this time, when the intelligent mothers began to notice how other mothers may have been involved in their children's condition, various manifestations of resistance around feelings of personal guilt often revived.

This was perhaps the most critical part of treatment, and the mother who was able to sustain her participation at this juncture without resorting to excuses about pressures of scheduling and the like, was well on the road towards achieving a more effective therapeutic relationship, with a beginning willingness to see the child's needs in context with her own wishes. These mothers became capable of articulating feelings which were often couched in terms of descriptions about the child's problems in school and with other people rather than about the child's problems with the parents, since readiness to cope on this level is often a later development.

Striving to open lines of communication among the group member helped them to develop insights, permitted open expression of ideas and feelings, and encouraged the disclosure of feelings of hostility, anxiety, and love.

An ultimate goal of the group leader was to see the mothers striving to resolve problems through participation with their family as a unit in programs, projects, trips, and activities.

The Leader-Therapist. In leading a mothers' group, a worker skillfully encouraged involvement and sharing, identified issues for more careful exploration, or solicited a reaction to a point. She also attempted to make available accurate information about the illness by occasionally inviting an allergist to the meeting. Mothers were thus able to gain a clearer understanding of the physiological aspects of the illness, what transpired during an attack, the role of medication and of diet, and other concepts of basic health care.

Many mothers had never had a meaningful explanation of the course and treatment of asthma. Offering this information in an objective, sympathetic manner also helped to provide psychological support. Helping them to understand that asthma could be affected by many things, including emotions, aided in cultivating a constructive attitude in which both overindulgence or rejection of the child could be avoided.

Under the critical eye of their supervisor, and medical and psychiatric consultants, the worker-therapist filled a vital role. They offered information, rendered support and assistance, encouraged self-expression, and stimulated discussion by posing penetrating questions and generally opened a portal of understanding between parents and children on the role of the family and home in the illness process.

Periodic Tests

Spirometric tests were taken periodically to measure change in pulmonary function. In addition, data were collected weekly from the mother's health index charts on attacks, wheezing, sputum, and medication. Follow-up testing was conducted after the children had been attending the clubs for three, five, and seven months.

Findings

The findings were significant. Fifteen out of 19 children in three groups for whom comprehensive records were available, showed significant increases in their spirometric readings (FEV^1), which pointed to increased lung capacity, ease of breathing, and generally improved pulmonary function. The other four children, while not achieving increased spirometry readings, showed greater responsiveness to medication. Almost all had fewer attacks of shorter duration and of less intensity. The increased spirometry scores averaged 10.67 per youngster—ranging from 8.25 for those in the group program for three months, to 9.04 for participants for five months, to 11.6 for those involved in the program for a period of seven months

Social Change

In the beginning of the program each youngster's social adjustment was evaluated on the basis of a psychosocial interview, and upon preselected criteria related to his participation with his group. Data in six specific areas were sought: first, on the child's ability to acclimate to group life; second, on his ability to relate to peers; third, on his ability to accept others; fourth, on his ability to handle feelings; fifth, on his participation in the group program; sixth, on his self-confidence. An evaluative scale plotting the early assessment of the participant's strength with a low of 0 and a high of 6 in each of these areas was devised.

At the termination of the program, each participant's social adjustment was again evaluated to determine movement, if any. The average change on a scale of one to six was 4.21 per participant.

An astounding finding in the experiment was the near-perfect correlation between the improved social adjustment of the individuals as revealed by the increased social index, and their increased spirometric readings (see Graph 1, p.69). These increased readings appeared in the main to correspond to the length of their participation in the group program.

The following additional results were discovered: youngsters with the lowest initial spirometry readings achieved the most significant improvements. In other words, the children who were the sickest achieved the most dramatic improvements. Patients ill for the longest time likewise attained significantly increased spirometric readings. It was also discovered that healthy patients (those less sick) became progressively healthier.

While a great deal of additional research is required—perhaps with larger samples, greater numbers of participants, and closer monitoring and control of data—the initial results of our study have already elicited much interest and excitement at the several pediatric, obstructive lung disease, and medical and psychological conferences at which they were reported.

Implications of the Hadassa Study

What does the Hadassa experiment appear to tell us?

The results of this modest experiment seem to have far-reaching implications which may offer us some additional insights into the complexities of intractable asthma, as well as considerations towards a rehabilitative approach to the illness. Features that should particulary occupy our attention in considering newer treatment modalities for the asthmatic child are:

1. The efficacy of the small social group as a medium for treatment and for effecting change;
2. The close correlation between improved social adjustment and increased pulmonary function;
3. The feasibility of the treatment of intractable asthmatics

CORRELATION OF SOCIAL AND SPIROMETRIC CHANGE

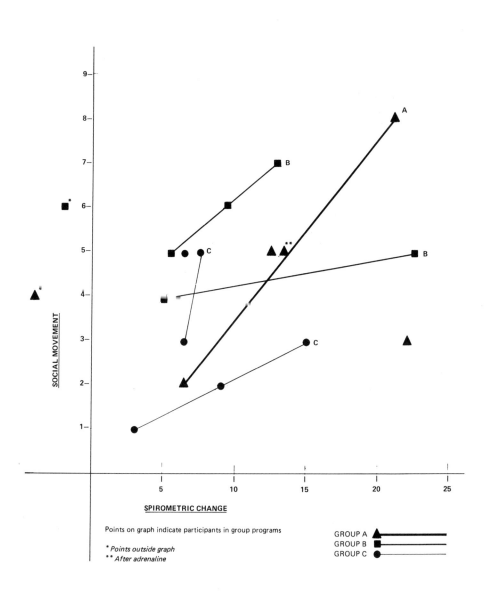

Points on graph indicate participants in group programs

*Points outside graph
**After adrenaline

GROUP A ▲
GROUP B ■
GROUP C ●

in small social therapy groups as out-patients, rather than through institutionalization;

4. The potentialities inherent in working with mothers (and fathers, too, if available) and their children toward achieving improved social functioning and, it is hoped, an attendant reduction in asthma symptomology.

8

THE SMALL GROUP AS A MEDIUM FOR TREATMENT AND CHANGE

Why the Group Setting?

Man's social hunger—his need for acceptance, to be part of something larger than himself—has been noted since time immemorial. His yearning for social contact and group experience date back to his early childhood.

A child is born into a family. As he becomes cognizant of those around him, his nuclear, or immediate family gradually grows to include grandparents, aunts, uncles, and cousins. The expanding, so-called associative circle is one which for most individuals, continues to enlarge as he grows older, to include playmates, schoolmates, and friends.

Group contacts provide support and encouragement through the establishment of relationships which in turn offer opportunities for one to test reality, and to learn about onself as a person. Group participation can have a profound impact on the development of attitudes, norms, and patterns of functioning. It can provide opportunities for a person to gain a better perspective of himself by seeing himself in contrast to others; to experience reality, to verbalize, and to express feelings.

The child who has been deprived, frustrated, or rejected, or the child who feels anxious, fearful, insecure, or inferior because of a physical limitation, is often hampered as a result of his disability, and may find it difficult to establish effective social relationships. Such a child shows his social maladjustment in a variety of ways. He may be aggressive and appear threatening to other people; he may be submissive, autistic (withdrawn), or hyperkinetic (over-active). Sometimes he is fantasy-laden and far away from the world of reality.

Few children are born as social problems. The majority become misfits as a result of unbalanced diets laden with heavy doses of rejection, frustration, and deprivation. It is not uncommon for children to be caught up in some of the parental needs discussed in earlier chapters. Denial of approval also helps to create social misfits, as does emasculation by overprotective, demanding, or pampering parents. Equally, children may be conflicted, or exploited, rejected, and deprived by parents, siblings, or by others.

The supportive social therapeutic group, which is in effect a miniature community, a small social system, can help in the modification of a battered self-image.[70]

The Group Method

Dreikuss, a pioneering psychotherapist, observed long ago the enthusiasm of his patients when he introduced the group method. He noticed that when he discussed with a group of patients case histories and incidents which no one except the patient himself was aware of, others expressed their opinions readily and "even the most reluctant were drawn into such a group."[71]

Conveying Points of View

Dreikuss felt that through the medium of the group "one could convey points of view to patients which they would never have permitted to be presented to them." He found it of interest too that the impersonal attitude of other patients had a disciplinary effect. "The goal directedness of all action," he observed, "could be clearly established, so that one was able to gain insight . . . "[72]

Removal of Feeling of Uniqueness

As a result of participation in, and through the medium of the group, Dreikuss felt that a patient could better understand what was of concern to another, rather than what merely concerned him alone. The "collective therapy" setting which ensued seemed to remove a feeling of uniqueness of personal problems and deficiencies. Patients in the group also appeared very frank and more depersonalized than they would have been as individual patients.

Knowing Oneself Better

S. R. Slavson, another pioneer in psychotherapy, relates that he came upon the efficacy of the group through progressive education, and social group work, and was impressed with the support and sharing of experiences which appeared to take place within this setting. He writes, "The characteristics and life style of a patient are shown with emphatic clarity in the course of collective [group] therapy . . . in the joint discussions with several other patients, each learns to know himself better, because he is able to learn from his observation of the others . . . "[73]

The Group As An Agent For Achieving Better Functioning

The group was seen as the ideal locus for an individual not only to reveal the nature of his conflict and maladjustment, but also as a medium to offer corrective influences. "Since man's problems and conflicts are recognized in their social nature," Dreikuss observed, "one must keep in mind that the individual as a social being is primarily concerned with finding his place in the group." To the person who has been engulfed or denied his individuality, this feeling of belonging is essential for social and emotional well-being. It permits the endurance of all hardships and adversities. Being a social isolate could be tragic. Dreikuss expresses it thus: "Not belonging is the worst contingency man can experience. It is worse than death."[74]

Emotional Isolation and The Group

The group is a particularly vital instrument today, when rivalry and a spirit of "each man for himself" prevails in much of society. Slavson feels that "the highly competitive atmosphere of our civilization produces a state of emotional isolation for everybody." Most people guard their real feelings. "Revealing oneself as one is," he writes, "entails the danger of ridicule and contempt. However, in the therapy group," he notes, "this danger is eliminated. For the first time the individual can be himself without fear or danger. This is an utterly new experience, and counteracts the basic fears and anxieties that are usually concerned with personal failure and defeat."

Social Adjustment and The Group

The social therapy group is almost a quasi-family, which, though providing reassurance and support, does not really demand an individual's ultimate commitment. As such, it is the ideal setting for social adjustment. Slavson finds that the group "provides subtle but all-pervasive encouragement for each member. It permits an unrestricted feeling of belonging without necessary personal bonds or attachments . . . it is truly a feeling of human fellowship without any ulterior motives of personal benefits or advantages . . . Accordingly," he says, "the desire to help each other in the group, springs from the deepest source of human empathy and fellowship—from a feeling of solidarity."[75]

The social therapy group has come a long way since Dreikuss's and Slavson's pioneering work, yet its fundamental purpose today remains very similar, and its value as meaningful, as when it was initially introduced nearly four decades ago. The group has become an important medium for social change as well as an important therapeutic tool. The shared interest in the group and the social function it plays, in addition to its therapeutic values, was seen by Ruitenbeck, who observed a number of positive effects of group experiences: "Groups are not only therapeutic, they fulfill an important social function." He commented, "People can share their anxieties and possibly become alive again."[76]

The Isolating American Culture

Our impersonal society offers little compassion for the individual with special needs. It is inherent in our system that recognition is accorded to the successful person, people who are different are overlooked or isolated. Our technological society is also frequently dehumanizing: it places man against the machine, and sets up achievement as the sole criterion of success. In the process, sensitivity, feelings, and human worth are put aside. These features of our existence plus the highly competitive American culture, many feel, encourages facade building. The American is trained not to reveal himself or his feelings. "The successful man who has had his expertise validated by his peers," Yalom writes, "too often strives to protect his public image at all costs. If he has doubts about his adequacy, he swallows them, and maintains constant vigilance, lest any personal uncertainty or discomfort slip through."[77]

The system which encourages one to hide his real feelings is seen by Yalom as "isolating" and "crippling," since it "curtails communication not only with others, but with oneself." The put-on facade which man needs to perpetuate his self-image, becomes so necessary that "in order to eliminate a perpetual state of self-incrimination for personal dishonesty, the successful individual comes to believe in the reality of his facade, and attempts through unconscious means to ward off internal and external attacks on his self-image . . . "

In the small social or therapy group, these restrictive norms are changed. There is no need to maintain a facade. The person is encouraged to experiment with openness. There are risks in disclosing thoughts and feelings, but when others are non-judgmental, one is generally accepted rather than rejected. When the individual sees others similarly possessed of doubts and fears, the process is self-reinforcing.

A Response to Self-Alienation

What happens to the child who has become alienated as a result of difficulties in adjusting?

Karen Horney sees self-alienation as a defensive device which the child develops as a response to basic anxieties originating in lack of harmony in parent-child relationships. When parents, because of their own neurotic conflicts, are unable to see their child as a separate individual with needs of his own, the child "uses energies which would usually be devoted to his self-actualization" just to survive. Such an individual attempts to differentiate between his "ideal self, his potential self, and his actual self." The person who attempts to shape himself in the form of an idealized but unattainable self feels self-hatred when there is a discrepancy between the idealized and the actual self.

The individual with a neurotic defense (which is often the case with the disabled child), is frequently frozen into a position and not open for learning. Horney sees this individual as "not striving to grow, merely to survive." Through the use of defense mechanisms he withdraws, attacks the environment, or himself.[78]

Argyris observes that the troubled person who finds it difficult to adjust, [becomes] more closed and less subject to influence." The more closed the individual becomes, the more his adaptive reaction will be controlled by his internal system. "But since his internal system is composed of many defense mechanisms . . . the behavior may eventually become compulsive, repetitive, inwardly stimulated, and observably dysfunctional, with the individual becoming more of a 'closed' system.[79]

In other words the troubled individual, if left to his own, tends to strengthen his defenses rather than have these modified by accurate perception. Consider how helpful the group can be to such a person.

Unlearning Old Patterns and Learning New Ones In the Group

"Therapy groups are as much or more concerned with helping patients to unlearn old patterns," Jerome Frank feels, "as they are with helping them to learn new ones,"[80] In the therapy group, therefore, the individual can hope to not only acquire greater interpersonal competence, but also to achieve the removal of maladaptive defenses.

The warm, understanding leader can help one to open up his secret world, to reveal his fantasies and his hostilities and to show his area of vulnerability. The leader and the group can also help him to appreciate his strengths and give him the confidence necessary to accept himself.

The Dynamics of the Allergy Group

A careful analysis of the development of the small social therapy group shows many of the features discussed in operation. There are roughly three stages, from the group's beginning, incipient state to the time it is able to become an effec-

tive instrument for the self-actualization of the individual,
capable of offering him the support necessary to fulfill his potential.

First Stage

The earliest stage sees the individual becoming oriented to
the other members and to the goals and purposes of the
group. Members during this period are in the process of evaluating each other, as well as the leader and the group.

Since individuals are preoccupied with being accepted,
those who fear nonacceptance may develop on a conscious or
unconscious level a defense against their real or supposed nonacceptance, which may find expression in their deprecation or
rejection of the group.

A striving for identity or similarity as a common denominator also characterizes this stage. For the asthmatic youngster
(or parent) this need is partially fulfilled by a common disability and affiliation with the "allergy club." This shared interest often tends to accelerate the process of individuals relating to each other, and also tends to expedite their subsequent
acclimation.

Second Stage

In the next stage of development, members who have generally gained a certain measure of acceptance feel free enough
to react, to complain, and to offer personal criticism. The
abandoning of social conventions, and the tension which is frequently engendered, is useful for the therapeutic process. It is
at this stage, that members of both the mothers' and childrens' groups are able to raise issues, to discuss conflicts, to
take issue with the leader. Through this ferment they are
aided to begin to assume a greater role in the resolution of
their own problems.

The small social group, which has aspects supplementary to
the pure therapy group, can. bring out much feeling through

the medium of skillfull programming. For example, a puppet performance in which the youngsters act out not only their own roles, but those of their parents as well, can afford an opportunity to articulate and to share a particular conflict situation which one might not be able to otherwise express until much later.

The varied programmatic elements, the games, trips, arts and crafts, and drama activities, also offer the group leader an opportunity to observe members in various situations that may be close to the reality of their everyday existence. This feature can serve to expedite the advent of the third stage, which is characterized by a sense of group cohesion.

Third Stage

It is at this stage in particular that a strong feeling of intimacy and closeness prevails. There is an increase of warmth and greater trust between individuals, which results in the development of a feeling of confidence, making possible increased self-disclosure, and a more conscious effort by members to mutually assist in the resolution of apprehensions and problems.[81]

What the Group Can Achieve

The group can help to achieve a variety of objectives for the client. How does acceptance, trust, and group support help the individual with problems? Carl Rogers, one of the world's leading psychotherapists, sees the process actualizing assistance as follows:

The patient becomes free to express his feelings.
The patient begins to test reality and achieves more discriminating feelings of himself, his experiences, his environment and of other people.
He becomes increasingly aware of the incongruity between his experiences and his self-concept.

He becomes increasingly able to experience without feeling threatened the therapist's positive regard for him, and to develop his own feelings of self-regard.

He becomes less concerned about his perceptions of others, and their evaluations of him, and more about the effectiveness of enhancing his own development.[82]

The Role of the Group Worker or Therapist

Rogers sees the therapist acting as a "facilitator," creating the conditions suitable for "self-expansion." In the process the client is helped towards self-exploration, and begins to consider feelings which were previously denied awareness.[83]

The individual gains acceptance not only from the therapist but from the group members. The group setting is seen as an especially meaningful and vital experience in effecting change. Rogers feels that for the individual it achieves acceptance by peers, rather than just by the therapist, as is the case in a one-to-one setting—acceptance by others who are not paid to listen, who don't have to care.

It is this contact and acceptance by others which is vital to achieving "good validation," which many patients have been denied in their childhood and while growing up. It is especially essential today, when the extended nuclear family, which in the past had often helped a person to find in it at least someone to extend "acceptance," or to give validity to a personality, that has virtually disappeared. This acceptance by others is almost a critical necessity for good mental health in a society that "appears bent upon dehumanizing the individual, and dehumanizing our human relationships."[84]

What Changes Occur to the Individual in the Group

Rogers sees the following happening to the individual within the group:

In regard to feelings and personal meaning, he [the client] moves away from a state in which feelings are unrecognized, unowned, unexpressed. He moves toward a flow in which ever-changing feelings are experienced in the moment, knowingly, and acceptingly, and in which they may be accurately expressed. The process involves a change in his manner of experiencing. Initially he is remote from his experiencing. An example would be the intellectualizing person who talks about himself and his feelings in abstractions, leaving you wondering what is actually going on within him. From such remoteness, he moves toward an immediacy of experiencing, in which he lives openly in his experiencing, and knows that he can turn to it to discover its current meanings . . . in general the evidence shows the process moves away from fixity, remoteness from feelings and experience, rigidity of self-concept, remoteness from people, impersonality of functioning. It moves toward fluidity, changeness, immediacy of feelings and experience, acceptance of feelings and experiencing tentativeness of constructs, discovery of a changing experience, realness and closeness of relationships, a unity and integration of functioning.[85]

In effect, then, the client comes into better contact with his feelings, develops a greater openness, and becomes more understanding and accepting of himself.

When this occurs, Rogers believes that he "moves away from perceiving himself as unacceptable to himself, as unworthy of respect . . . toward a conception of himself as a person of worth, as a self-directing person . . . with the frequent result that he develops much more positive attitudes towards himself."

Attitudes about his own person that were in the main negative, more often than not become positive. Rogers continues,

The patient becomes more open to his experience of himself and of others . . . he becomes more realistic . . . he improves in his psychological adjustment . . . his aims and ideals for himself change so that they are more achievable . . . the initial discrepancy between the self that he is, and the self that he wants to be is greatly diminished . . . tension of all types is reduced—physiological tension, psychological discomfort, anxiety.[86]

The changes which occur during therapy are, according to Rogers, noticeable not only at this time, but later too. He notes, "Careful follow-up studies conducted six to eighteen months following the conclusion of therapy indicate that these changes persist."

Our impressions would tend to concur with his observations. In the following chapters we observe the impact of the group experience on a number of representative asthmatic youngsters.

9
SELECTED CASES

Introduction

The five cases presented on the pages which follow are representative of the asthmatic youngsters who, with their parents, have been members of our allergy clubs in recent years.

The children and parents in these programs were referred by their physicians and allergists, who continued, throughout the course of their participation, to oversee and to monitor their patients' medical treatment and progress.

The setting is a suburb of New York, although the concept and program utilized for these groups is based upon the Hadassa Hospital experience which is described in Chapter 7.

To a large degree these youngsters and their mothers have much in common with their Israeli counterparts: intractable asthma, which is unresponsive to conventional treatment, concern over adjustment and functioning, and environmental problems which tend to create for them situations of stress and conflict. They also experience similar apprehensions over their feelings of hostility, self-esteem, social isolation, and identity (See Chapter 3).

They too have been able to a greater or lesser degree to avail themselves of the group, the quasi-family setting comprised entirely of children suffering from asthma to help work through their socialization and rehabilitation needs, and to find more appropriate ways of resolving their conflicts than those which appear to be contributing to their asthma symptomology.

The method employed in working with them is essentially social group work, which, like other therapy approaches, seeks to provide services to promote the children's healthy and sound functioning. The unique feature of the small social group approach, in contrast to the pure therapy group, is that it attempts to see the individual not only from a psychological perspective, but also within the broader social dimensions of his existence; i.e., within the context of family, peer group, school, and community.

Since it is within these environments that problems of functioning and adjustment most frequently occur, the process seeks to view the remediation of the client's social, emotional, and physical health needs from these contexts as well.

The cases presented here concern typical problems of intractable asthmatics, all of a complex emotional nature—disturbed patterns of family relationships, overdependence, repression of feelings, parental manipulation of children, and vice versa. One may observe conditions which create the loss of an individual's social role, and which serve to engender feelings of social isolation, a poor self-image, loss of identity, and powerlessness.

The leader-therapist seeks in each instance to identify the stresses and patterns within the individual's various environments which appear to manifest themselves in an exacerbation of asthma symptoms and which seem to give rise to the recurrent chronic bronchial asthma condition. He then seeks insights into the meaning of the dynamics of the symptoms, and tries to provide corrective experiences to prevent social breakdown, to provide rehabilitation where breakdown has occurred, and to foster more appropriate ways for the patient to express and to resolve his conflicts.

As the group finds an identity of its own, members begin to plan activities based upon their interests. When this occurs, the group begins to become a more effective vehicle for reinforcing existing strengths and partializing disabilities. The dynamic force of the group as an agent for change can be seen in several instances. The group process helps to avert pathology and dysfunction—and strives to develop awareness, a sense of responsibility, and an improved self-image that grows out of new-found social roles, which bring with them a consciousness of the problems which are creating stress. Through collective support the group thus becomes an agent for the individual to achieve identity and to reach his potential. It continues to develop and to help fulfill individual needs, and in several cases to achieve an improved level of social functioning. In our experience with the asthmatic child, this also helps to promote improved health functioning.

THE SETTING

The setting consists of several small social groups comprised of 6 children each ranging in age from 6 to 13. All have chronic, intractable asthma, and are in the main unresponsive to medication. Their attacks vary in frequency, intensity, and duration, and their condition impedes their physical functioning to varying degrees, causing frequent school absences and requiring repeated hospitalization.

As a result of their debilitation, the children are apprehensive about their daily routine, which continually emphasizes restrictions such as reduced physical activity and limits on travel, which might take them away from needed medical help. To reduce anxiety, and to prevent their coming into contact with allergic substances such as pets, pollen, smoke, and foods, they likewise have been cautioned to avoid new, threatening, or provoking situations, or settings different from the routine and familiar. As a result, their contact with peers if often limited as well.

The children are seen regularly by an allergist, whose office serves as the meeting place for their group. The group meets weekly for sessions which last approximately one hour. On occasion, activities are held outside the office. Their mothers meet simultaneously in a separate setting with another trained social group worker.

The program is predicated upon a conviction, shared by an increasing number of health and behavioral professionals, that there is growing evidence of the influence of parental and environmental relationships on the emotional state of these youngsters, which in turn is closely related to their physical functioning and asthma symptomology—frequency of attacks, wheezing, and so on.

The purpose of the children's allergy club is to utilize the group process to enable the participants to achieve better functioning through supportive treatment and resolution of conflicts; to assist in their socialization in a nonthreatening, accepting environment; and through a comprehensive therapy program including both verbal and nonverbal activities, to provide reality testing to enable them to gain reassurance and support, to build their ego, and to help resolve and reduce stress and conflict which may be related to their health problem.

JANE: THE ABANDONED CHILD

Jane is a tall, robust nine-year-old girl who is in the third grade. She is attractive and has pretty features. Her mannerism is decidedly masculine.

She was born in a small town in Louisiana, where her father was a student at a local university. Her mother, a registered nurse, returned to work shortly after her birth, at which time Jane was placed in the care of baby sitters.

Jane began school in the south, where she completed first grade. At the conclusion of the school year, she and her mother, who is now divorced, moved into the home of her elderly maternal grandparents in a suburb of New York, where they lived for almost two years. They were living there while Jane was in the group. They have just relocated to their own apartment.

Jane has not seen her father, who left for Mexico after the divorce, since age three. Communication between them has been virtually nonexistent until recently when he made some effort to contact her.

Health Data

Jane's medical records show that she is an highly allergic child, sensitive to pollen, dogs, and various foods. She has had eczema intermittently since age one.

Her first asthma attack took place when she was two and a half years old, shortly before her parents' divorce. Since that attack she has been hospitalized for asthma eleven times, each admission lasting from four to seven days. Her condition has become progressively worse, and as of late there has been little response to medication.

The Group Worker's Report

Interview with Jane. Jane appeared for our first interview dressed in an attractive pants-suit. To conceal the patches of eczema at the creases of her elbows, she tried to keep her arms folded. She appeared ill at ease, highly anxious, and reluctant to speak.

I mentioned to her our plan to form a club comprised of allergic children who would get together each week to participate in activities and programs, and to share feelings about their illness. She appeared interested.

To make her feel more comfortable and relaxed while we talked, I asked whether she would like to work on an arts and crafts project with me. She nodded in assent. I proceeded to show her how we could make a "membership badge." I had arranged several pieces of precut wood, as well as alphabet noodles, paint, paste, and pins, and I began to assemble the letters for my own name and glue them on to the wooden base. Jane followed suit, hesitantly. We talked while we worked.

She wanted additional information on the club: what they would be doing, and who the other members were. I replied to her question, and mentioned that the identification tag would help us and the other members to get to know each others' names at the first meeting.

I asked Jane to tell me a little about herself. She told me that she and her mother lived with her maternal grandparents in a nearby city, and that she sleeps on a folding chair-bed in her mother's room.

She mentioned that her parents were divorced, and that her father, who she hadn't seen in six years, lived in Mexico. I asked whether she had any recollection of him, and she replied that she hardly remembered him since she was very young at the time he left.

I inquiried about her grandparents. She replied that she spent little time with her grandmother, because the latter was always busy doing housework. On occasion, though, her grandfather took her "places." In addition to Jane, her mother, and the grandparents, an aunt lives with them. Jane appears to resent her aunt.

There are no children her age on the block. When the weather permits, she plays ball and other outside games with a six-year-old boy who lives nearby.

I asked her whether she was friendly with any children from school. Her reply was a rapid "no." She does not invite any of her classmates to her house, nor does she ever go to theirs.

We continued on the subject of school. Jane dislikes school, especially reading and math. Even though she completed her first year of school in the south, it was necessary for her to repeat it when she moved north. She is therefore a year older than the others in her class. Her favorite activities in school are gym and recess.

She never reads for pleasure. She spends most of her free time watching television, even eating dinner in front of the TV set.

I asked her to tell me what she does on Saturdays and Sundays. She said that she generally stays around the house. Sometimes she goes "somewhere," or does something with her mother.

By this time Jane had completed her pin, which I admired approvingly. I asked if she would like to play a game with me, and she said "yes." We began to play the word game "spin and spell," which is somewhat similar to Scrabble.

After a few minutes of play, I noticed that Jane had difficulty forming words. She asked that we stop playing. I changed to "Dots" and "Battleships," paper and pencil games which require no verbal skills. She played enthusiastically, obviously enjoying herself. As we played, I tried to engage her in further conversation. She pleaded, "Please, let's just play," and "Let's stop talking."

At the conclusion of our interview, I told Jane that I was glad to have gotten to know her, and that I looked forward to having her in our new group. I told her that I thought the others would like to meet her, too.

Interview With Jane's Mother. Mrs. W. is 32 years old, a registered nurse who currently works at a New York State hospital. She is outgoing, attractive, blond, and seductive.

She relates that she worked hard to support her student-husband, whom she now despises. She left him because he refused to assume any responsibility for his family, and was more concerned with his books and student activities than with his wife and child.

Mrs. W. returned to work only a few weeks after Jane's birth because they needed the money. Between her work and household chores, she had little time to devote to her child, who was left in the care of a series of baby sitters.

She and her husband quarrelled often, usually over petty matters. After their divorce Mrs. W. asked him to stay out of Jane's life. Since then contact has been limited and infrequent. The father occasionally sends Jane picture postcards, but Mrs. W. discourages the child from responding.

Her parents, with whom they now live, are elderly and have little patience with Jane. Mrs. W.'s mother was recently hospitalized for diabetes, and her father was operated on a short while ago for a vascular condition which required corrective surgery. To the extent that it is possible for him to do so, the grandfather tries to fill Jane's need for a male figure. For example, at the beginning of the school year he took Jane to a father-daughter party at school. But Jane is really too much for him to handle.

Mrs. W. works full time, and is too exhausted when she comes home to spend much time with Jane. She tries to get away alone now and then for a weekend. Arguments between Jane and her grandmother are especially severe during the times that Mrs. W. is away. The disagreements usually relate to the grandmother's intolerance and impatience with Jane. During a recent weekend when Mrs. W. was away, Jane had a full-blown asthma attack which required her hospitalization.

Jane has been feeling particularly bad lately. It was discovered recently that she is sensitive to dog's hair, and consequently had to give away her pet dog. Jane was very much attached to the dog, and she misses him terribly.

The Group

A week later Jane and her mother joined the program. During the initial meeting, Jane manifested neurotic behavior and found it difficult to relate to the others in the group. She kept going to the bathroom for "drinks." She was anxious and unsure of herself. During the crafts part of the session, she kept telling the leader that her project (a papier-maĉhé animal) would never turn out as well as those of the other children. She was uncertain how to act toward the others, and was pointedly silly and giggly. With appropriate support, she seemed to progress well with her project. She works quickly and well with her hands. During game time, she continued to "act out" in a rough and tumble fashion, although considerably less then she did at the beginning of the meeting.

At subsequent sessions, as she began to gain confidence, she volunteered to guide us in a new crafts project—making piggy banks—and offered to provide the plastic milk containers needed. Later she took to helping others with their work.

Activities involving verbal or math skills continue to present difficulties. Jane's spelling is weak. She writes b's for d's and p's for q's. She finds it almost impossible to keep score for a game. She has trouble with basic addition, and is totally lost when it comes to long division, which her class is now learning.

During successive sessions, Jane has become more open and communicative with the other members. She shared the news with the group about a phone call from her father in Mexico. Though the shock of hearing from him precipitated an asthma attack, she was glad that he had called. She also told about an exchange with him of mail and Christmas gifts. She commented, "I'm happy to know that I have a father, even if he is in Mexico."

Recently she made a two-day trip with her mother to Canada to get a new medication. Upon her return, she told the group about her travel experiences, and how nice it was to be able to sight-see and to be on "vacation" together with her mother.

Assessment

The medical records show Jane to be a very sick child. It appears that Jane's unfulfilled need for love, acceptance, and self-esteem, are basic factors relating to her emotional and physical condition. From early childhood she has been a victim of a succession of rejecting events. She has failed to develop a sense of security, attachment, and rootedness so vital for the emotional well-being of a child. Dating from infancy, her mother left her in the care of others, and neither she nor her father had time for her.

Her parent's divorce, which apparently was attended by much unhappiness and discord at home, reinforced her feelings of rejection, as did her father's subsequent departure for Mexico. What little security she could derive from the knowledge that she had a father, through the occasional postcard exchange, was halted by her mother who, in the process of punishing her former husband, was in effect hurting Jane.

The return to the north again reinforced Jane's feelings of rejection. Moving in with grandparents, who had neither the health, patience, nor energy to cope with an energetic youngster, did little to fill her need for acceptance and security.

There is very little verbal communication between Jane, her grandparents, and her aunt. Jane resents her lack of privacy and the makeshift sleeping arrangements, and probably holds both her mother and aunt responsible for her having to sleep on a folding chair-bed.

She has been living in virtual social isolation, and though she is starved for social acceptance, she is not quite sure how to handle herself with others. There appears to be little family solidarity in her grandparents' home, where even dinner is an individual activity. She is not comfortable or secure enough to bring friends into the house. She has been separated from her dog, which she came to love, and which had given her a bit of security.

Jane's mother's frequent weekends away are disquieting and frightening, yet Jane cannot share these feelings with her mother for fear of losing her love and being even further rejected. The grandmother appears to transfer her resentment about Mrs. W.'s trips to Jane.

Jane's self-image is exceedingly poor. She is embarrassed by her eczema, which she tries to conceal. Being required to repeat first grade served as a further blow to her self-esteem. Her problems with math and language skills reinforce her feelings of inadequacy, and continue to identify her in her mind as a failure.

Jane's Attitude Toward the Allergy Club

Jane was apprehensive about joining the allergy club, but willing to give it a try. During the initial sessions, she seemed to carry over her sense of failure and lack of self-worth to the area of friendship. She experienced difficulty in relating to peers. (She had chosen to play with a young neighborhood boy rather than attempt to form associations with classmates.) Though eager and alert, she appeared uncomfortable in the group's social setting, and expressed her insecurity by her giddiness, frequent trips to the bathroom for drinks, and acting out.

She uses her hands rather skillfully when working on crafts, but shows her lack of confidence and low self-esteem by such remarks as, "Mine isn't so good," and "Yours is better." She keeps testing to see whether the leader and other members of the group really accept her. Though uncomfortable and resentful of the worker prying into her life during the early sessions, she seems to have accepted her and is beginning to relate more easily to her, as well as to the other group members. She is gradually finding friendship and acceptance, and is becoming a contributing member of the group. Through her giving, she is also receiving strength and recognition.

Mrs. W.

From the initial reports of the parents' group meetings, it appears that Mrs. W. has a great many conflicted and ambivalent feelings about her daughter, alternately loving and rejecting her. On the one hand she wants to do what is best for her child and help her in her illness, yet she regards her as a "ball and chain" keeping her [the mother] from her own independence.

Attractive, with her own social needs, and concerned about her disappearing youth, through her interaction with the other mothers she is coming to understand that she feels restricted and limited by Jane, particularly by the child's illness. She is anxious and confused about herself as a mother. She is also bitter toward and resentful of her former husband, who fathered a child for whom she now has sole responsibility. In initially discouraging correspondence between Jane and her father, she was manipulating the child to sever contact with him. She is reluctant to allow him to enter the child's life and to perhaps share some of the responsibilities, preferring instead to punish him, herself, and the child in the process.

Intervention and Desired Outcomes

Jane needs a great deal of support and acceptance. She is angry at her mother, but afraid to show it. She is inquisitive about her father, but apprehensive that closer contact with him will annoy her mother and cause the loss of her love.

As the mother learns to understand her own feelings, and the needs and feelings of her child, she will begin to see her role in Jane's illness more clearly. With appropriate counseling and support from the parents in her group, Mrs. W. is coming to understand her own involvement, and is beginning to move toward a more accepting and supporting position.

Perceptible Changes—Several Months Later

A number of noteworthy changes have begun to emerge in both Jane and her mother's life patterns after several months in the group. Mrs. W. and her daughter have moved into their own apartment. Jane now has her own bed and her own room, for which she has helped select the decorations and furnishings.

Mrs. W. has come to realize the importance of her daughter having friends. In addition to her membership in the allergy club, Jane has joined the Brownies, and Mrs. W. tries to include one of her Brownie friends or classmates in some of their weekend plans. Recently she invited a friend from school to sleep over. Mrs. W. has also started to engage herself with Jane over the weekends, and is spending more time doing things with her: going apple picking, skating, and taking short trips to places of interest nearby.

As the mother has moved closer to an understanding of Jane, she has also begun to take note of the factors which seem to exacerbate her child's illness. She has become more conscious of her daughter's capacity for involvement in physical activities before she begins to wheeze or to have an asthma attack. As a result, she has been able to balance Jane's activities, varying those that are physically demanding or taxing with those that are more relaxing.

Reestablishment of contact between Jane and her father was recognized as potentially important. Mrs. W. has agreed to assume the initiative in writing to her former husband and suggesting that he have an on-going relationship with the child, which could be useful. This shows considerable maturation and movement on her part. Jane's father has called and written a number of times. Though Jane was overwhelmed by the initial contact (as noted earlier, she had a severe asthmatic attack the first time she heard his voice), a sustained relationship with her father can give her much needed support.

The need for remedial help for Jane in language and math skills has been suggested to Mrs. W. Overcoming disabilities in this area will further improve Jane's self-image and aid in bolstering her ego.

Jane's continued presence in the group is having a positive influence on her. She relates to the worker and feels accepted, as evidenced by her growing ease with the worker and her increased ability to articulate and to communicate her feelings more freely. She is beginning to develop a sense of belonging to the group. She has made friends and is working on relating to them in a more normal, and less neurotic, manner.

She is being given opportunities in the group through crafts, games, drama, and other activities to show her strengths and capabilities, and is in the process of building her feelings of worth and self-confidence. This is a beginning step in the process of socialization, which a successful group experience with her peers will hopefully reinforce.

Group participation seems to be helping Mrs. W. understand herself and her child fully, and to see the relationship between her child's emotional well-being and her physical condition. Simultaneously Jane is being reinforced by her mother's understanding, and by the support of her own group, which can provide her with much needed feelings of security and acceptance, and can help her toward a success identity. As this happens, Jane will hopefully become not only a happier, but also a healthier child.

Peter: The Confused Boy

Mrs. K. is an intense, neurotic woman in constant motion, who uses tranquilizers to "keep calm." She suffers from peptic ulcers and an assortment of other ailments. She is also highly allergic to a number of foods.

This afternoon she appears particularly upset. Her day started with a bout with her son Peter, aged 6. It was her turn that morning to serve as aide at the nursery of four-year-old son David. In addition, during the course of the day she would have to shop for and prepare supper for company that was expected that evening, arrange several carpools, and straighten the house. In between, she and her son Peter were in for the weekly meeting of their respective therapy groups.

In the Group

At the session, Mrs. K. reported that Peter had complained of a stomach ache the past Monday morning, and said that he did not feel well enough to go to school. Although the Monday-morning blues are a fairly regular occurrence at the K. household, she continued, "I took him to Dr. B. for a checkup." (Visits to the family doctor are not rare with Mrs. K., and it is an unusual week when neither she nor her children visit the doctor at least two or three times.) Dr. B. examined Peter carefully and said that he couldn't find anything wrong with him, and that he appeared well enough to go to school. "To be on the safe side," Mrs. K. continued, "he suggested that Peter's food be limited to liquids, and to light, easily digestible foods."

Mrs. K. dropped Peter at school, and told him that if he did not feel well, he should go in to see the school nurse and ask her to call home. She continued, "No sooner did I get home, but the telephone rang, and it was the school nurse informing me that Peter was in her office. Peter told her that he did not feel well, and that he had my permission to go home. The nurse said that Peter would like me to come to school right away to pick him up. Since I had a number of stops to make, I picked Peter up first, and decided to take him shopping with me at the mall.

"When we arrived at the mall, Peter complained that he was hungry. We went into a nearby restaurant and Peter wanted to order a frankfurter and French fries. I told him that Dr. B. had said that he could have only liquids, or soft, easily digestible foods. Peter said that his stomach ache was all gone, and insisted that I get him a frank and French fries. When I hesitated, Peter raised his voice, and started shouting that he was hungry. I was embarrassed that people would think that I was cheap, so I succumbed to his pleading—but instead of getting him his first choice, I ordered a grilled cheese sandwich for him, and then, remembering what the doctor said, an orange drink. Peter was only partially satisfied and complained that he was still hungry. So I bought him mashed potatoes."

Mrs. K. wanted to know from the other mothers whether she had done the right thing. They explained that she had committed a number of basic errors, which appeared to be reinforcing Peter's neurotic behavior.

The Monday-Morning Syndrome

The group discussion continued along the following lines. It should have been fairly apparent to Mrs. K. that Peter was not very anxious to go to school on Monday mornings. The reasons, they speculated, could have been any one of several—after a relaxed Saturday and Sunday, when Peter could do as he pleased, and when he had his father and mother largely to himself, he obviously preferred to extend the weekend rather than return to the regimented classroom.

What awaited Peter in the classroom? the therapist prompted. How competent a student was he? How understanding were the teacher and the students about his physical condition? Was he capable of competing with the other kids scholastically, or in athletics? How did it feel to be left out when teams were being chosen, especially since everyone knew that Peter was the first to get out of breath, and that when he did he made strange wheezing sounds.

The other mothers and the therapist tried to help Mrs. K. piece it all together. Once the doctor had pronounced Peter fit to go to school, should the mother have planted a seed of doubt in his mind as to how healthy he was by suggesting that he see the nurse if he did not feel well, and that she should be called to take him home?

The mothers continued to speculate and to question: was Peter being rewarded for his "illness" by being driven to school rather than commuting by bus with the other children as he generally did? When the child called from the nurse's office, shouldn't the nurse's opinion have been sought? If he was not well enough to stay in school, should his mother have taken him shopping, or should Peter have been brought home and made to rest in his room for the afternoon?

While his mother believed that she had acted properly in denying Peter the franks and the French fries which he wanted in favor of the grilled cheese, did Peter see it this way, or did he view himself nevertheless as being rewarded by having another favorite food out in a restaurant? Assuming that it was necessary for his mother to take him shopping, might she not have minimized the treat atmosphere by giving him nothing or providing him with merely a drink, and explaining to him firmly why he could not have anything else? Should the mother have allowed herself to be embarrassed into succumbing to the boy's desires?

Peter's Manipulations

After a series of similar encounters and discussions it became apparent to Mrs. K. how she was being manipulated by her very clever six-year-old, who knew precisely how to get his way, and had trained his mother to respond to his wishes. It was suggested to Mrs. K. that she be firm with Peter, and anticipate his apprehensions about going to school on Monday mornings. The therapist explained that in addition to the factors cited, it was conceivable that Peter was wondering what good times he was missing when he went off to school, leaving his four-year-old brother home with mother. What kind of fun was he being left out of?

To offset his curiosity, it was suggested that the mother point out the responsibilities of each person in the family: the father, who left each morning for work at the plant in order to earn money for the family's needs; the younger brother, whose responsibility it was to attend nursery school, (and the mother was to proceed to describe what the nursery program was like, and how it too challenged the capabilities of a four-year-old); and the mother, whose chores consisted of cleaning, cooking, shopping, food preparation, etc. Mrs. K. was to tell Peter that this was pretty much the routine that the family followed on Monday, Tuesday, Wednesday, and on other weekdays.

The mother was told to avoid extending privileges to her younger child while Peter was away, and instead, if a treat such as a candy bar was to be provided, to obtain two, and to hand them out to both children when Peter returned from school. Peter was thus reassured that there was little to be gained by staying home rather than going to school. He was further assured that any kind of reward or favor intended for his brother would be equally shared with him.

Peter's Father

On another occasion Peter's father visited with the parent's group. Mr. K., tall and good-looking, is henpecked and withdrawn. Whenever he attempted to speak, his wife would invariably interrupt to offer the "correct version" of whatever was being discussed. After several minutes it became apparent how Mrs. K. perceived her husband.

Timid and self-effacing, Mr. K. could assert himself only in limited spheres of family life. His wife was the one who made all of the major decisions. Even in regard to his employment, it was she who decided that her husband should change his original job for a position which she considered more "glamorous," insisting that it was her intention to make "something" out of him. Her husband's parents were not permitted to visit the K's home. To quote Mrs K., "They are kooky people"—and her husband was in turn discouraged from visiting them.

At subsequent sessions Mrs. K. related that she and her sons spent their summer vacations at her parent's bungalow. Her husband remained in town, visiting them on occasional weekends. Mr. K.'s input to his sons' development is minimal. While he is somewhat of an athlete, during his weekend visits

to the bungalow he spends the bulk of his time playing ball
with other men, rarely with Peter. In the city Mr. K. occasionally plays ball on the block with Peter who, as Mrs. K.
puts it, "must take his turn at bat like all the other kids who
gather around whenever his father comes out to play with his
son."

Mr. K. described one of the infrequent outings that he took
with Peter. The trip was to a major league baseball game, one
of the really rare occasions when Peter had his father almost
entirely to himself. Almost, because several of Mr. K.'s friends
came along.

Indulging Peter

Mr. K. told of indulging Peter, and responding to his frequent nudgings by purchasing things for him each time the
vendor came by: two hot dogs, soda, popcorn, and peanuts.
Finally he told Peter that he had reached his limit, and would
make no further purchases.

Outside the stadium, on the way home, they passed a
souvenir stand. Peter asked that they stop and look, and insisted that his father buy a pennant for him. The father refused, recalling the various treats that he had already pur-
chased for him, but Peter was adamant. The father tried to
hold firm, but when Peter started making a scene and calling
him stingy, the father gave in "to avoid being embarrassed in
front of my friends."

It didn't take the group long to figure out that Peter had
learned to manipulate his father as easily as his mother.

Assessment

During the intensive therapy sessions which ensued, considerable time was spent in helping Mrs K. sort out her feelings
about her husband. She told of her own childhood, in which
she was constantly able to manipulate her parents into getting
what she wanted; of her dates; of a lengthy courtship with a

prospective suitor whom she turned down when she realized that he was "too strong" for her and could not be dominated. Mr. K. was an ideal mate; he was weak, and had been effectively emasculated in his childhood by rigid parents.

Insecure and Confused

Mrs. K. continued to play the dominant role. Her behavior carefully covered up her own insecurities, which became particularly apparent to her after Peter's birth. She lacked confidence in her capabilities as a mother, she was unsure how to handle Peter, and would fall to pieces at the onset of illness. Each ailment became a crisis, with her husband unprepared to cope and herself uncertain about how to handle it.

Even fairly routine matters were handled in confused and ambiguous ways. For example, in regard to determining a suitable bedtime for Peter, Mrs. K. had been vascillating between letting him stay up as late as he wanted, or opting for an early bedtime. Did she involve her husband in trying to establish a suitable time for Peter to be in after play? "Well, after supper when Peter is out playing ball for a couple of hours his father will lamely suggest that perhaps it's time for him to come in, that Peter 'should consider' getting ready for bed. Peter argues, disregarding his father's urgings, and remains outside as long as he can.

"He even ignores his mother," the father relates: "even when she comes out and yells, he doesn't pay much attention to her." It is only "when she screams at him at the top of her lungs and threatens to pull his hair out," that Peter finally "drags himself in."

Peter in the Group

Peter and his mother have been in therapy for 6 months. The child has been guarded, cautious, and uncommunicative. His association with the others in the group has been limited. At first he tried to manipulate the children into getting his

way, but there was too much resistance. He tried several times
to bully the group into giving in to him, but likewise with
limited results. Peter began to notice that the methods which
he had successfully used on the "outside" were not working
too well with his peers.

For a while, he withdrew into himself. This is not too sur-
prising, considering the confused pyschological environment
from which he comes. Many activities which appealed to others his age hold but lukewarm interest for him. He gravitates
toward athletics and is particularly fond of bowling. The therapist, who is aware of his capabilities in this area, has attempted to schedule bowling as a group activity from time to
time. Here is an area in which Peter could display his skill in
a socially acceptable manner and receive appropriate recognition from the group. At a bowling session which was later arranged and attended by his younger brother, David, he took
special pride in teaching some of the others how to bowl.

He is slowly gaining in tolerance for others, and is beginning to accept people as they are, without trying to manipulate them only in his own interest. But he still demonstrates
difficulty in making decisions. In view of his family environment, his lack of decision-making ability is not too difficult to
understand.

During the winter, Peter and his parents were at a Miami
motel for a holiday. Following a day of many activities, a day
far too strenuous for a child of his age and capacity, Peter had
a full-blown asthma attack shortly before midnight. Though
he was obviously in need of medical help, and his parents
were aware of excellent medical facilities available nearby,
they could not decide whether he should be taken to the hospital. Six-year-old Peter was called upon to make the determination. Though Peter opposed going, when the attack persisted for several hours more, his parents finally decided that it
was necessary to bring him to the hospital. By the time they
arrived there, he was in severe status asthma.

The child has come a considerable distance during these
past months. He has become more communicative. He is
friendlier, and is gaining a sense of security. He is in the process of working out his feelings toward his younger brother,

and is beginning to accept involvement with others on terms which are not always dictated by him.

Mother's Growing Understanding

Through her participation in the therapy group, his mother is beginning to understand Peter's (and her own) problems more readily. She is becoming increasingly aware of her conflicted feelings toward her husband: her desire to dominate him coupled with resentment over his weakness, which leaves her with the bulk of responsibility for making the decisions in their family's life. She and her husband are also beginning to be helped to recognize how their conflicts are affecting the child. They are also in the process of examining the effect on Peter of the poor male image his father presents him.

The group experience has encouraged Mrs. K. to build up her husband instead of knocking him down. Together they have begun to strive for firm and sensible approaches in raising Peter. They are beginning to consult with each other on basic matters regarding the child in an effort to arrive at a consistent approach in relating to him. They are, in brief, trying to let Peter know exactly where he stands with them, and how they feel about basic issues.

So far, the results are encouraging. Peter finds less need to manipulate, and interestingly enough, as he has begun to find his home situation more stable and secure, the incidence, frequency, and intensity of his asthma attacks have been reduced considerably.

Terry: The Ugly Duckling

Terry is tall for a thirteen-year-old. She has long, black wavy hair and a pretty face which is distorted by edema (fullness) resulting from the heavy doses of steroid medications which she takes for her asthma. She currently takes eight cortisone pills every other day, in addition to Marax four times daily.

Terry is from an affluent family. Her father is a corporate executive, and her mother, a school teacher. The family lives in a comfortable suburban home with a swimming pool, and owns three late-model cars.

Terry's asthma began two years ago, when she was eleven. The youngest of three sisters, she is overshadowed by Mary, eighteen, a bright, attractive freshman at a New England college, and Nancy, a shapely sixteen-year-old who aspires to be a model.

Terry's Illness

Terry, an eighth-grade honor student, is absent from school almost as often as she is present. She is afflicted by almost constant wheezing and frequent asthma attacks, which last a day, two days, or longer. She keeps her prescriptions handy and medicates herself. Her mother has been taught by Terry's uncle, a physician, how to administer adrenaline, but when the girl is unresponsive to the adrenaline, she must be rushed to a nearby hospital for emergency treatment. Terry has been a patient at the hospital so often that she knows most of the staff by name. She comments, "I feel very comfortable there [at the hospital], and I am not particularly anxious to come home."

Terry is an unhappy child. She is not well enough to participate in physical activities in school, and though she enjoys walking, if she covers any significant distance, she is left wheezing and breathless. She cannot ride her bike around the block without losing her breath. On the occasions that she uses the family pool, she does not swim, out of fear of becoming winded, nor does she paddle, perform strenuous exercises, or put her head into the chlorinated water.

Family Background

Terry has few friends, and she wonders why those that she does have put up with her, since, she says, she loses her temper so quickly. Her middle sister is a difficult act to follow. Terry says, "Even though I hate to admit it, Nancy is beautiful," and she is quick to add, "She spends most of her time making up." Her oldest sister, Mary, who comes home from college occasionally on weekends and holidays, is kinder to her than Nancy, and easier to take.

Her father, Mr. O., works long hours at his firm. He leaves for his office early in the morning and returns late at night. His job is demanding, and when he gets home in the evening, he has neither time, energy, nor inclination to be with Terry. Whatever spare time he does have is devoted to a local civic club of which he is president. He previously was chairman of a regional fraternal order. Though Terry believes she could be close to her father, she finds that he is far too busy to pay attention to her, and even when they are together she feels that he does not really listen to what she is saying. She also regards him as being totally under her mother's control.

Terry's Mother

Terry's mother is a tall, large-framed woman. Mrs. O. is a hard, domineering, and rigid person who speaks openly of her disdain for her child. "Terry was unwanted," she relates. She had preferred to have only two children, and Terry was an accident. The mother never accepted her, nor has she forgiven her for causing her middle-aged spread, the weight she put on during her last pregnancy, which she has been unable to shed. She is sensitive not only to her figure, but to the fact that she passed her fortieth birthday a few years ago, and is desperately attempting to hold on to her youth. The mother has been teaching kindergarten for the past ten years. During Terry's infancy she preferred to be out of the house, so she arranged for a maid to take care of her children while she returned to work.

She believes that Terry's illness is "put on," and that she could control it if she really wanted to. "She uses her asthma to make our life miserable," she fumes, "and I won't put up with it and let her ruin our lives. Terry made it so that we

could not go on our vacation three times last year. I told
Terry on many occasions that if she persists in being bellig-
erent, and continues to have attacks, I would have her put
into a strait jacket, and sent away to a mental institution."

Terry's Suicide "Attempts"

Terry is despondent. She recognizes her mother's antipathy
toward her, and has on several occasions contemplated suicide.
During her most recent attempt, she picked up a carving
knife, placed it against her chest, and told her mother that she
would stab herself if her mother did not change her attitude
toward her. Her mother relates, "I knew she wouldn't do it;
she loves herself too much to commit suicide. Yet I fear that
she may some day injure her sister Nancy."

Terry was referred to the allergy group by her allergist, who
advised the mother flatly that he would refuse to continue
treatment unless both mother and daughter would go for psychological help. They had seen a therapist briefly previously,
but the mother discontinued the visits, feeling that they were
not making any headway.

Terry's Feelings of Rejection

Terry and her mother have been part of the program for
two months. Tense and anxious at the beginning, Terry is
gradually beginning to open up. She is bright, understands the
source of her own emotional turmoil, and is perceptive about
her mother's feelings toward her. She offers repeated illustrations of her rejection. "When I'm ill at school, I go to the
nurse's office. I never call my mother," she relates. "Once,
when I had an attack, and I called my mother, she started to
yell at me over the phone." Her most serious attacks follow
big blow-ups with her mother or middle sister.

Asthma as a Weapon

Terry is aware that her asthma is a powerful weapon. "My
mother gives in to me when we have a fight, because she is af-

raid that I will have an attack." Terry takes her mother's
threats to institutionalize her seriously, but says that she will
never consent to being "sent away."

She is aware of how "upsetting" her illness is to her family,
and to her mother in particular. She is terribly conflicted,
basking in the attention the illness gives her and alternately
hating herself for her asthma. She says that she is determined
to "make it" in spite of her mother. "If only she wouldn't be
so cruel to me." She illustrates, again to the others, "My
mother knows that I am allergic to cigarette smoke, yet she in-
sists upon smoking even on the way to our sessions. When I
protest, she counters, 'It's my car, and I'll do as I like. If you
don't like it, you can get out and walk.' "

Terry feels that the only one in the family who understands
her is her oldest sister. Her father is capable of understanding,
but he is weak and dominated by her mother.

Mrs. O. has been attending sessions reluctantly. She is annoyed that she must come each week since there in "nothing
wrong with me," and the illness is "Terry's problem." She
spends the bulk of her time at the sessions sulking and re-
counting what a miserable child Terry is. She "tunes out"
when members of the group attempt to question her about her
own feelings and behavior. It is only with a great deal of effort
that she allows herself to see her daughter's side of the problem. "She is just an ungrateful, miserable child." She offers an
illustration: "several days ago I was taking my class to the circus, and we had a few extra tickets. I invited Terry to come
along. You would expect that she would be appreciative, and
grateful: instead she was hostile, and insulted me in front of
my fellow teachers."

Terry's and her mothers versions of this, and several typical
incidents as discussed at their respective groups, follows:

Terry's Version

Feelings. My mother is not at all concerned about my feelings and the things that irritate me. She thinks nothing about
smoking in the house or in the car though she knows that the
smoke aggravates my allergy.

The Circus. My mother doesn't care at all about me. I don't think that she really wanted to take me to the circus in the first place, but it happened that she had some tickets left over because some of the children couldn't go, so she took me.

It's a long trip into the city, and the circus lasted several hours. We had a long wait in front of the circus afterward for the bus to show up, and then a lengthy trip back to the school where my mother teaches. When we got there, I was tired and irritable, and feeling awful.

Mother knew that I wasn't feeling well, but do you think she cared? She found some of her friends and stopped to chew the fat with them, when she knows how awful I was feeling, and that I wanted to get home.

So I said, "Mother, please let's go home now," and she just stood there gabbing away like mad with her friends as if I didn't exist, and told them that I just wanted to get home to watch my soap operas.

About Her Attractive Sister. Nancy is much prettier than I. I think all of the medication that I'm taking is disfiguring my face. [Terry is on steroids.] My sister Nancy either makes fun of me or just ignores me. On Thursday I asked her to lend me her top, which would have gone nicely with a plaid skirt that I was wearing, but she wouldn't, even though it was just going to lie there in the drawer . . . Then Saturday night everyone has something to do except me. I don't even mind that too much, but I like to be with people too.

There I was sitting in the living room watching TV, Mother and Dad were getting ready to go out!—*they're always going out!*—and Nancy is primping and teasing her hair because she knows that Fred is coming over. Well, finally Mom and Dad are almost ready to leave, and Fred comes, and everybody tries to shove me back in to my room out of the way, and I'm not going to let them push me around. So I said, "I'm not going!" Mother knows by now that there is no point in starting up with me, because when I get provoked, I can have an attack. But do you know what happened? Fred's a nice guy. I don't know why Nancy is so lucky to have him interested in her. Well, anyhow, he invited me to play with them, and then after a while I left them and went back to my room to watch TV.

Mrs. O.'s Version

Feelings. Terry is just plain insolent!

The Circus. She embarrasses me in front of my friends all the time. For example, last week, after taking her to the circus, for which she didn't show an ounce of appreciation, I stopped to chat for a few minutes with my friends. Terry rushed up to me, and says, "Mother, I want to go home, and *right now.*" She put on such a scene that I had to apologize to my friends for her behavior.

About Her Attractive Sister. She hates her sister Nancy [who is three years older than Terry] *with a vengeance.* She constantly gets in Nancy's way, and interferes with her life. I think she's just plain jealous of Nancy's good looks, and the fact that she's attractive and has boyfriends.

Saturday night, when Nancy had her boyfriend over, she asked Terry to let her use the electronic game, which is connected to the TV set that Terry was watching in the living room. Terry has a TV in her own room, but she plunked herself down in the living room, watched TV, and refused to move.

We were on our way out for the evening to have dinner with friends. Even my husband, who has the patience of a saint, was provoked and about to let Terry have it. But I stopped him, and told him to leave her alone. If he had hit her, and she had had an attack, it would have ruined our plans, and we wouldn't have been able to go out. Finally Nancy's boyfriend solved the problem. He suggested that Terry play the TV game with them—and she did. I guess she likes him and is willing to listen to him. I understand that after a while she went back to her room and left them alone.

Notwithstanding the huge chasm between them, Terry and her mother have in a limited way gained some knowledge about themselves, and have begun to communicate with each other.

With "appropriate support," Mr. and Mrs. O. were able to get away to the Caribbean for a long-sought-after weekend vacation, during which time Terry remained at home with Nancy. In spite of the anticipated fireworks, the sisters managed well. Nancy was especially accommodating, perhaps because she was visited several times during the weekend by her boyfriend, who also found time to be friendly toward Terry. During the weekend, Mrs. O. called to find out how the sisters were managing. She told Terry that she was calling her long distance at considerable expense, "just to speak with you." Terry was impressed that her mother thought enough of her to spend a lot of money to call her from so far away.

Mother Begins to See Herself

Terry's mother has begun to see how and why her child uses her illness. She is perhaps somewhat neurotically gratified by her daughter's total dependence upon her when she is ill. She says, "When Terry is ill, I am extremely compassionate to her." She is also gradually beginning to recognize her biases in favor of her middle and older daughters, and is starting to explore her own frustration, resentments, and intense conflicts over the child.

Terry's condition began to improve somewhat for a while, but then took a turn for the worse. Mrs. O., who had begun to see more clearly her role in her daughter's illness, has resisted vehemently being identified with her condition. She is closed to any effort to probe or to examine her motives, her favorite expression being, "My daughter is the sick one, *not I*."

Termination

For the past several weeks she has been building toward termination of her association with the program. As the process of her own involvement in her daughter's condition has become more painfully apparent to her, she has desperately sought a face-saving reason to leave the program. Recently she alluded to the fact that her husband was experiencing financial difficulties, and that she has sensitized her children to the need to eliminate any unnecessary expenditures.

Terry has become conflicted over her responsibility to help her father in his financial need, and feels trapped because her continuation in the group, her major source of understanding and acceptance, may be concluding. Recently, she indicated that she did not know whether she would be able to continue in the group much longer.

Terry is no longer in the program. Her mother called to inform the receptionist that "Terry has decided to discontinue her sessions," and that notwithstanding the mother's "best efforts" to convince her to remain, her daughter would not be continuing in the program any longer.

Fred: The Emasculated Boy

Twelve-year-old Fred has been an asthmatic since infancy. He is handsome but frail looking, as a result of frequent bouts with his illness.

The history of his ailment, especially during the past five years, has revolved around intense attacks followed by extended periods of hospitalization. During the brief respites in between, his wheezing is so bad that he is confined to bed most of the time.

Though he is bright, with above-average intelligence, Fred was out of school over 100 days last year. After a day or two back in school, it is not unusual for him to be absent for the next week or two. The emotional strain of being far behind in his studies is overwhelming.

An ardent scout who has earned his eagle badge, Fred's image of himself was low, compounded by his inability to attend troop meetings. His frustration over being unable to join others in his troop for overnight hikes, outings, and other activities, has progressively seen his ties with scouting—his main love—weakened. As a result of his illness and his limited association with his peers, he has gradually lost the bulk of his friends. To make matters worse, he developed acute eczema, which gradually spread from his legs to his elbows, arms and face. He looked as bad as he felt, and his appearance was enought to drive away his few remaining friends.

Family Background

Fred is the youngest of three children, third in line after an attractive, bright, and talented sixteen-year-old sister, and a fourteen-year-old problem-laden brother.

Fred's Mother

His mother, a real estate broker, maintains an active office in suburbia. She is a slightly built, hard-looking woman approaching forty, an only child of a devout church-going mother who read the Bible to her daily, and a hard-drinking father who was a "man about town."

Mrs. J.'s memories of her early childhood years, which were spent in the Midwest, lack precision. She does not recall exactly why, but at the age of five she was boarded out to a neighboring family for about a year. She surmises that it may have had something to do with her father and "the law." She remembers the neighbors she lived with as being extremely cruel and insensitive to her. She next relocated to the Southwest, moving in with a relative, and shortly thereafter rejoined her mother.

An asthmatic herself, Mrs. J. traces her condition back to the period when she was first separated from her family. She vaguely recalls that both before and after the separations she and her mother protected each other from the cruel world about them, and especially from weak-willed men who couldn't be trusted. The similarity between these men and her father, who rejoined the family a year or two after her return, is striking.

After being reunited with his family, the father, a heavy drinker, made several attempts to "go dry." but was unsuccessful, and returned to the bottle. Mrs. J. recalls that he spent many nights away from home, and frequent battles between her parents regularly followed upon his return. She remembers also his physical debilitation and degeneration brought on by his excessive drinking and the effects of advanced venereal disease.

During her teens Mrs. J. was forbidden to go to movies or parties. It was only when she attended college away from home that she began to go out with boys.

Marriage to Mr. J.

Shortly after her graduation, she met Mr. J. Several years her junior, he was easy going, good natured, and her inferior intellectually. Since he was prepared to accept her word as law, they were soon married. He suited her "just fine."

Prior to joining the asthma parents' group, the J.'s had been seeing a psychiatrist in regard to their older son, and marriage counselors about their sexual incompatability.

Mr. J. is a jewelry salesman. His wife regards him as immature and irresponsible. "He can never hold on to a few dollars," she complains. "Would you believe it," she asks, "he once went in to an auto showroom and ordered a car and accessories without even asking the price?" She points to a cabin cruiser that he recently acquired in the face of their inability to financially carry it, as further "proof" of her husband's irresponsibility regarding money matters. Mr. J., who comes from a family of strong females, is conflicted over his need to be dominated and his desire to prove his masculinity.

In a replay of her parents' experiences, and of her mother's feelings about carefree, untrustworthy men, Mrs. J. shows her disapproval of her husband in the most obvious way that she can, by denying him sex. "I can't understand why people get so excited and worked up about sex," she rationalizes.

Fred's brother is severely disturbed, and has been receiving psychiatric treatment for a number of years. His sister, a strong-willed replica of Mrs. J., is thriving. Trapped between feuding parents—a strong mother and a weak father—Fred has become their football. His conflicts are expressed in his very serious asthma.

Two Years Later

Two years in the parents' club have helped Mrs. J. to understand the similarity between the family patterns of her own childhood and those of her current situation. She has become aware of the motives behind the selection of a husband whom she can dominate, and has begun to see how she has been manipulating him sexually. Mr. J., who now has a better understanding of what has been happening, has begun to assert himself more. His wife, with considerable reluctance, is beginning to allow him to participate in decision making, and their sex life is beginning to improve.

Through his participation in the allergy club, Fred has gradually been gaining confidence in his abilities, and his image of himself has begun to improve. He does not see himself as being particularly frail or sick. In a setting where asthma is the common denominator of all members, becoming winded when participating in vigorous athletics is not unusual. Nor is a patch of eczema, a fairly common sight, a cause for embarrassment.

Fred has been able to open up, and to articulate long repressed feelings about himself and his family. The group process has been a useful medium in helping him to sort out his anxieties and fears and to achieve increased self-awareness. A talented craftsman, he has created some beautiful items for which he has received recognition. He has assisted others in various aspects of design and construction of their projects, which has given him greater confidence in his capabilities and has helped lessen the negative image which he has had of himself.

The home scene has improved considerably. His father has begun to emerge as a respected male figure, and the mother's domination has been tempered. As the climate at home has begun to change, and the amount of conflict and friction reduced, Fred's health has shown dramatic improvement. The confidence gained through his participation in the group has been reinforced by a commensurate reduction of hostility at home. Hardly anyone now needs to manipulate the child.

Fred's condition has continued to improve. He is attending school with greater regularity and has developed some new friendships. He has flown by himself to and from Florida to spend a holiday with his grandmother (something that his mother would never have considered allowing him to do previously). He has begun to take up his old loves, scouting and the outdoors.

His bouts with asthma are gradually becoming a thing of the past, and his eczema has almost cleared entirely too.

Amy: The Child of a Frightened Mother

Amy, who is now eight years of age, has been part of the allergy group program for two and a half years. Though considerably shorter than other children her age, she is pretty, vivacious, and loving, and above all, she is today in relatively good health.

Almost ready for discharge from the program, she has come a long way in the last 30 months. From an average of 50 to 60 absences from school each year, and 8 to 10 hospital admissions for status asthma and collapsed lungs, heavy dependence upon steroids and other medications, Amy has averaged 5 days out of school this past year for routine children's illnesses, has had no asthma attacks or hospitalizations and is now relatively free from medication.

Amy's parents are both cultured and well-educated suburbanites. Her father is an administrator of a large school, and her mother, a supervisor of records at a municipal office. Her sister, who is five years old, is pretty and verbal.

Diminutive Amy had considerable apprehension when she joined the program. Her wheezing and coughing were almost constant. Her asthma history went back to age three, shortly after her sister was born, when her mother observed in Amy what she described as "difficult breathing." Amy is allergic to a long list of things, including foods, pollen, mold, dust, and pets. Her parents, apprehensive about her condition, had during the next few years made the rounds of doctors and clinics for the "elusive magical cure," which they were unable to locate. Their allergist thought that the group program might be worth a try.

Interview

A diagnostic interview of the child and her parents, at which time a comprehensive psychological and medical history of Amy was obtained, served as the basis for her assignment to an appropriate allergy club. The interview utilized play therapy, and included work on simple crafts projects—the construction of a membership pin made of a small strip of painted wood to which alphabet soup letters spelling out her name were affixed and a clasp added. Amy was informed that other members of the club, which would begin meeting shortly, would be wearing similar identification tags at the initial session.

Amy In the Group

At the first meeting several weeks later, she was introduced to group members, her peers in age and health. All were wearing membership identification tags similar to hers. A warm and accepting therapist put her at ease and made her feel comfortable. She was told that the club's program was to consist of talking, activities, and games which would incorporate suggestions of the children with those of the therapist. She was told that she did not have to participate in the group activities unless she cared to. She was likewise not required to speak or to get involved in group discussions unless she so desired.

At the beginning her groups' programs centered around simple crafts, with the youngsters talking while they worked on various projects—a cork doll, pipecleaner animals, mosaics constructed from different-sized and colored peas and beans, painted stone paperweights, clothespin memo holders—which required a minimum of artistic or craft skills.

Amy's lack of self-confidence was apparent. She constantly compared her work with that of the other children, commenting that their abilities and achievements were far superior to hers. Amy's initial hesitations about undertaking these projects were sympathetically heard and gradually overcome by the worker, who encouraged, supported, and praised her achievements. As Amy's confidence increased, she participated a bit more readily, and gradually began to undertake newer and more complex projects.

The amount of conversation which took place between Amy, the other children, and the therapist at the early stages of the group was minimal. At successive sessions, specific activities were introduced by the leader to afford members greater opportunity for expression. Upon her suggestion, the club built a small frame stage, and undertook to construct a number of hand puppets.

The Puppets Speak

Under the therapist's direction, the puppets served to articulate many feelings which Amy and the other children could not otherwise express. Amy's puppet told what it felt like to be left alone inside a classroom on a cold or windy day when other children and their teacher went to the playground outside to play. It told the story of parents fearful for the life of their child, and wracked with emotional turmoil each time the symptoms of an acute asthma attack began to appear. It told of urgent deliberations over a decision as to whether or not to rush the child to the hospital.

The parent puppets were often hesitant and unsure of themselves. Amy's would relate how it felt to be treated by strangers while in a hospital emergency room in the middle of the night.

Her friend's and her puppets told many stories which the youngsters could not otherwise bring themselves around to telling, annoyance over not being able to ride a bike, or to run like other children, what it was like to be constantly concerned about the ingredients of each food item that they were about to eat, lest a reaction be precipitated.

Group Activities

The club program featured many activities. In addition to puppetry and crafts, Amy played games and did exercises. Most of the games involved blowing—playing windball—a game in which members were divided into two teams who sat around a table, each member with a straw in her mouth. The object of the game was to score points by blowing through the straw at a ping pong ball with sufficient force or continuity to knock it off the opposite side of the table, in spite of the best effort of the opposite team to keep the ball on the table by blowing it back from their side.

Another game the children played was to try to blow out a candle from an ever greater distance. Though Amy was not consciously aware of the fact, the exercises sought to strengthen her scapular muscles, to help her and her friends develop the ability to abort an attack.

On occasion the members and leader went on a bowling trip, or to shop, or on excursions to places of cultural interest. In anticipation of these trips the children were required to plan, to help organize, to suggest programs—in short, to interact.

As Amy and the others became more secure, accepting, and comfortable with each other, conversation began to flow. The puppets were no longer the devices required to convey her feelings; she could talk about things openly and directly with the other children. She began to share with the others how it felt to be the older sister, and to see attention lavished on a younger sister, how Mommy and Daddy quarrelled often, and how difficult it was for them to make up their minds about things . . . How Mommy not only worried about her (Amy's) health, but how she was terribly concerned that maybe something was wrong with Daddy, and how she and Mommy worried over Grandpa, who was in and out of the hospital with some kind of heart condition.

Amy's Involvement With Others

Amy would listen to the others speak of their apprehensions and concerns and would react, offer her opinions and suggest solutions to their problems just as they would for hers.

Slowly Amy came to recognize that life entailed a series of vicissitudes, ups and downs which every person seemed to experience. In many instances, it appeared to Amy and to her friends that all the bickerings and misunderstandings of parents seemed to come to an end when a child came down with an asthma attack. The child's illness seemed to be one of the few factors that brought parents together, and although subsequently there might be considerable recriminations as to whose fault it was, or who or what precipitated the attack, at least for the period of the attack the child was in the center, and her parents appeared to be together.

It was a new experience for Amy to be able to hear others tell how they felt about their illness and that they too had fears and concerns. It was normal to be frightened by attacks, but it was important to recognize that other children had attacks too—and that though they too were frightened, they survived.

The group was a safe place to talk about anything that bothered her—she could share her worries, for everyone had worries. Hearing from others in the group that they had conflicts with their parents, and feelings of rivalry and competition with their younger brothers and sisters, helped Amy think through her own apprehensions and recognize that she didn't have to feel guilty because she sometimes had bad feelings about her parents or her sister.

The therapist read stories and led discussions about being different, the theme often being that though one might be different—black or white, tall or short, with glasses or without—one was no less valued. Specific games selected by the therapist proved that on occasion there were benefits to being shorter than others. Eventually Amy no longer considered the title "Shorty" offensive.

The meetings offered empathy and support, and in addition to helping her gain confidence, they gave her a better understanding of herself, helping her to achieve better functioning. Amy was changing very gradually, and her new image was something that seemed to please her, and to make her a little happier.

Amy's Mother

At the same time that Amy was meeting with her friends in the allergy group, Amy's mother, a diminutive, attractive woman in her early thirties, was settling down for her weekly sessions with the mother's allergy group. She was a bundle of nerves.

The mothers' group moved into high gear much sooner than the childrens', and it didn't take too long for a variety of apprehensions and insecurities to surface. Amy's mother was tense and fearful that something terrible might happen to Amy one of these days. It was reassuring to hear that other mothers were similarly apprehensive over their children's asthma.

Amy's mother discussed the conflicts around her adequacy in mothering a "sick" child, and wondered how she could have enough time to devote to a demanding younger child and to simultaneously be a good wife.

Amy's father had recently been appointed to an administrative position at an academic institution, a demanding job which he apparently lacked the confidence to handle. His strained emotional and physical condition were added causes of concern to her. She worried also about her aging father's precarious health. He had been in and out of the hospital for a recurrent coronary condition, and his last attack had made him into a semi-invalid. She had a premonition that he would not live too long and she had fears and anxieties: whether she had been a good enough daughter, and to what extent she was responsible for his condition. She had her share of problems, worries and apprehensions, not least of which was Amy's debilitating and recurrent illness.

She discovered that the other mothers in the group had their share of problems. Listening to their concerns and reactions afforded her an opportunity to place things into perspective and to more clearly understand the source of her own strains. The group discussions focused on practical matters too. The mothers exchanged advice on how to prepare attractive meals for highly allergic children, how to bake wheatless cookies, and swapped recipes for other nonallergenic satisfying snacks.

Gradually Amy's mother stopped blaming herself for her father's poor health. She also began to see her husband's problems more objectively. She recognized how a stressful environment was contributing to her daughter's condition. As she came to understand asthma more clearly, she developed a more realistic and even optimistic feeling about her child's ability to lead a fairly normal existence notwithstanding her condition.

On several occasions her husband joined her in the group. Sometimes he posed a question about his wife's overconcern with illness; at times he expressed apprehension about his own health, and wanted to talk through his own stresses and strains, and to discuss his feelings of inadequacy.

A Happier and Healthier Amy

It is difficult to assess which of the family members were most positively influenced by their group involvement. It is probable that all were moving simultaneously. It may have been Amy's improved image of herself and the gradual reduction of the frequency and intensity of attacks, which was producing a healthier climate at home; or perhaps it was the security and confidence that the mother had gained, and the support which she could now offer the other family members, which helped inspire a feeling of confidence in her husband and children, to which Amy too so admirably responded; or perhaps it was a combination of these: the warmth and security which permeated the home and which made for a happier, less tense family situation which resulted in Amy's gradual improvement. No one will ever know for sure, but the fact is that 30 months after joining the group, Amy was a different child— far happier and leading an almost asthma-free existence.

10

Coping With Stress: A Life-Long Struggle

Gaining a Sense of Security

Is it possible to more effectively prepare a child to cope?

The child who has been helped by his parents from infancy onward to adjust to varying situations has the potential of developing a healthier approach to meeting life's viscissitudes than the child who has been left to shift for himself.

Childhood Stress

Stresses begin to occur early in childhood, and originate with the needs of the infant. In addition to food, sleep, and dry diapers, the child expresses through crying other needs which we may not always understand. At times the need may be for stimulation or security—to be picked up and cuddled, to have his position changed to a more comfortable one, or to find relief from boredom.

The child who does not receive a response to his needs, or appropriate stimulation when required, often withdraws and loses "eye-to-eye" contact with others rather than developing a sense of trust in people. Receiving sympathetic, positive responses and guidance enables the child to utilize his capabilities and to achieve self-esteem. The ability to cope with frustration remains as he moves from infancy to childhood. Security in relating and responding to others emanates from a feeling of certainty that a person has acquired early in life.

During each age period the child must be helped to function on his own level, rather than to fulfill unreasonable expectations of his parents or others. He must also be helped to learn to cope with unpleasant situations as well as with pleasant ones. The child who is helped to develop at his own pace and level and is made to feel that he is valued, and that his parents care about him, is gaining in emotional maturity and is being assisted in cultivating the potential to cope successfully with a variety of stresses that inevitably will beset him in the future. On the other hand, the child whose parents have been overly permissive or overly rigid in his upbringing, may acquire feelings of uncertainty, clinging to his parents and finding it difficult to adjust to new situations. Such a child may find that separation from his parents in order to attend school or for some other purpose, even for short periods of time, may be anxiety-provoking. Such a child's behavior may also reflect uncertainty, and possibly fear of school—if not to the physical facility, then possibly to the reactions of the teachers or of the other children toward him. He might also be wondering what is going on at home while he is away, and whether his parents will come to pick him up after school.

Other challenging situations with which the child is unprepared to cope may bring on similar expressions of apprehension or self-doubt. Some children show their feelings of apprehension to stressful situations by bed wetting, stuttering, nail biting, thumb sucking, or through physical symptoms: stomach ache, headache, or palpitations.[87] As indicated in earlier chapters, the chemical and psychological effects of specific or ongoing stress can, when the potential susceptibility exists, often manifest itself in a specific organ or part of the body that may be most vulnerable. In the case of about 3 percent of American children the manifestation is in the lungs or in an aspect of pulmonary functioning which may induce coughing, sputum, wheezing, and other symptoms representative of a beginning or developing bout with asthma—and which at times culminates in a full-blown asthmatic condition.

Adjusting to Life Pressures

The burdens of emotional pressures of various types affect us not only during infancy and childhood, but at all stages of life and under varying circumstances. We have observed that the body has its own way—emotional, chemical, and physical—of responding to demanding features of our everyday existence, which are or can be potentially irritating, dangerous, frightening, exciting, or confusing. Emotional stress, as we have seen, can be brought on by pressures, self-doubt, leaving a familiar setting, or by excessive or disturbing noise. It can even be prompted, as we have noted, by pleasant but stimulating, taxing, or exciting events or situations. Emotional tension and anxiety may result from factors present in the home or in our associations, studies, job, or in almost any other aspect of our environment.

While its impact is felt often, few people ever really learn to understand how this tension or anxiety affects them, and only rarely do they acquire the ability to learn how to live with it. However, as we have mentioned, if we are able to master stress, it can strengthen our resistance and prepare us for future encounters. But if we do not learn how to handle it adequately, it can gnaw at our minds and our bodies.

Beyond Childhood

Each period of our development appears to have its own unique form of stress. We have observed some of the stresses of infancy. The times of childhood and beyond also have as we have noted their share of frustrations and adjustment problems related to growing up.

Adolescent Stress

Following childhood, the adolescent years, beginning with puberty at about age 12, and lasting to age 20 or 21, are especially tumultuous and turbulent. This period is one of dramatic body changes during which time boys become men, and girls change into women. A fast-growing body full of surging hormones produces along with acne, new hair, and changed voice and fuller figure, significant biological and social stresses. Not only is it strange to learn to live in a changing body, but the awkwardness is compounded by the heightened social demands which are placed upon the adolescent. The shy and withdrawn, or the overacting youngster are both equally struggling for a sense of identity, and the acquisition of a perspective and a self-image.

It is a cultural phenomenon in Western countries that physically vigorous and active bodies are kept quiescent. Whereas in former days or in other cultures, many people were already working or married at this age, American society places adolescents in a "neutral world" somewhere between child and grown-up. There they are made dependent and treated like children, but expected to act like adults. The attitude of our technologically advanced society toward its young people is an inconsistent one. On the one hand it requires them to continue their schooling for extended periods, often into their twenties, to achieve skills and acquire technical proficiency; while on the other hand these demands cause adolescents to remain unmarried and usually under parental control for long periods of time. The ensuing conflict over submission to authority—being obedient to parents and teachers while striving for individuality and self-fulfillment—often places the adolescent who is seeking identity and trying to explore life on his own, in direct conflict with the adult society about him. Add to this pressures of parental expectations, and a desire on the part of some parents to keep the apron strings taut, to prevent the growing up and emancipation of their offspring—or consider the alternate approach of other parents who let their children strike out on their own and gratify their every desire rather than to defer these to later, and we begin to understand the elements that make up the constant, stressful struggle for identity and direction on the part of growing youth.

Adult Stress

The line differentiating adolescence from adulthood is indeed slim, since it is usually chronology rather than biological difference which separates the two. The period of adulthood has been called the middle years, and we find in them boundless opportunities for satisfaction, intertwined with many potentially stressful experiences. These are years of achieving on the job, or making a mark professionally; of marriage, raising a family, acquiring a home, becoming a member of a community—the period of settling in.

With it, however, come the potential vicissitudes of job satisfaction or lack of it; of pressures to produce and strivings for promotions; of receiving acceptance and satisfaction. It is a period of family changes, of births, with the attendant concerns of child-raising, and the financial pressures of providing for hungry mouths and for bodies that quickly outgrow their clothing. These years call for caring for dependents who require expensive education and who all too soon are grown up and off to school, frequently away from parents, out of town. It is a time of concern about money and material fulfillment, marital satisfaction, sexuality, and stability.

It is during this period that a harmony at home is sought that is often more idealized than real. It is a time for concern for health and illness, and the thousand and one ingredients required for adult adjustment and survival in a society which is crime-laden, competitive, plagued by a troubled economy and threats of nuclear war, and by relatively little concern for the welfare or dignity of the individual who often gets lost in the shuffle.

The older years bring further potential for bliss and stress: for satisfaction derived from achievement and success, and for disappointments, recriminations, and self-blaming for the less than ideal situation that an individual finds himself in. Health concerns, preparations for compulsory retirement, with its attendant societal and personal attitudes, are the major anxiety-provoking features of this stage . . . so opportunities for stress and their potentially damaging effect on our emotional and physical well-being remain with us virtually throughout our entire lifetime.

11

Helping the Asthmatic Child

What, if any, are the implications of the preceding pages?

1. A host of surveys and research papers on the causative factors of asthma exist.
2. It has become fairly clear that it is no single factor, but rather a constellation of factors, which appear to affect asthma.
3. These factors may operate independently or in combination.
4. Contributing causes vary in different people, and their impact, even for the same person, sometimes varies.
5. The illness is a common one, frequently frightening, and sometimes chronic and disabling.
6. Asthma is a complicated illness and there is much about it that is still unknown. What seems to be clear, though, is the close interrelationship between the functioning of the lungs, the central nervous system, immunological disorders, allergens, and infections.

7. We have seen the possibility of the presence of genetic factors, and the probability of a predisposition or vulnerability to the ailment.

8. There is considerable evidence about the impact of emotional factors, and of the close relationship which exists between the psychological climate and the social environment, of the asthmatics' physical functioning and the manifestation of his asthma symptomology.

9. A very close relationship exists between anger, fear, anxiety, and stress; and the manifestations of a struggle between overprotecting or rejecting parents and their child, who is attempting to construct an independent existence, have been noted, as have the physical reactions which all of these cause.

10. Asthma literature and research appear to support the contention that there is considerably more neurotic behavior on the part of asthmatic youngsters (and their parents) than among others. Though this appears to be the case in regard to most asthmatics, it seems particularly true for those suffering from intractable asthma. Ironically this feature of the illness tends to offer hope for its remediation. From our studies it appears that more than 60 percent of children suffering from intractable asthma are able to achieve a significant remission of asthmatic symptomology.

Predicated upon available information, it is our belief that efforts to treat the patient piecemeal are of little avail. The question of how to treat him in his entirety, and not just for his sickness, is for most physicians and behaviorists a challenging but rather remote goal. Few facilities exist for this type of team treatment and care, and while supported by many, the concept of team treatment is practiced by few. The need which we have attempted to cite is one which sees the individual patient receiving appropriate comprehensive medical and psychological assistance relative to his needs in his own environment.

We have suggested that institutionalization, the removal of the individual from his family and from familiar surroundings to an artificial setting, and his ultimate return to an unchanged original environment, is rarely the answer, and that the health village concept is too far off to be of practical value for those needing help now. Instead we have proposed treating both parents and children as out-patients at local hospitals, or in other settings within their own communities, with the assistance and cooperation of their physicians, allergists, and trained social workers or group therapists.

We have identified the small social group led by skilled therapists as a particularly appropriate setting within which to accomplish the goals of treatment and improved social adjustment. The Hadassa experiment, and a number of years of independent research and practice, appear to have confirmed for us that small therapy groups, with populations comprised exclusively of asthmatic children and their parents, can be an effective medium in a significant number of cases in helping patients to achieve increased socialization, self-confidence, and an improved self-image, which appear in turn to have, for many, contributed to the alleviation of asthma symptoms and to an apparent remediation of their condition.

The knowledge and information relating to factors contributing to the illness which have been gained can, we hope, be put to good use on behalf of the asthmatic. For example, a concern for improved socialization for the asthma sufferer need not be reserved for the group, but can be put into practice regularly in other settings. There are likewise other areas in which the sensitive parent, skilled physician, and trained therapist can help in remediation by identifying major contributing conditions and attempting to do something about them.

Physician, Therapist, and Parent

The Physician's Role

Select an internist, pediatrician, or preferably an allergist in whom you have confidence. If you are in doubt about his qualifications, check him out with your local hospital, medical society, or with your own family doctor. If you can develop confidence in your doctor, you will be spared the effort, anxiety, and heartache of having to seek the elusive doctor with the magic cure, who exists mainly in the minds of parents who do not have full confidence in their physician. Make certain that the physician is one with whom your child has rapport, and with whom he can identify in his efforts to get well.

The physician, in addition to assuming overall responsibility for the medical evaluation and treatment of the patient, can determine the offending allergens: what the child is sensitive to in the realm of food, clothing, plants, animal life, fumes, and atmospheric conditions. The allergist can do more than advise. In many instances, under a good regimen of medical care, he may be able to make the patient less sensitive.

The Therapist's Role

The therapist should be able to advise the parents on the stress factors in the child's world: his apprehensions, sensitivities, fears, anxieties, and other highly charged feelings which appear to impinge upon his condition. The therapist may also be able to help the child work through many of his concerns in this area—and may involve the parents in an examination of theirs. It is to be hoped that the therapist will be able to provide the parents with a better understanding, not only of the psychological ingredients which appear to be influencing their child's health, but also how the parents and others in the family in turn affect and are affected by the child.

The Parent's Role

Through skillful observation it is quite conceivable that you too may be able to identify and note your child's tolerance for various activities and factors which tend to aggravate his condition. You should, for example, be able to determine the amount of sleep he requires to function at his best level, and whether or how he reacts to insufficient rest or sleep, and to plan accordingly. You can and should note his endurance in the realms of physical activities—running, jumping, cycling, swimming, ball playing, and skating. Pay careful attention and make a mental or written note on how much of these activities he can endure before he starts to wheeze.

You can by observation determine other factors which may be affecting his condition—his tolerance to cold, snow, wind, or changing weather, including rain and sunshine, whether he is affected by seasonal changes, how he reacts to excitement, laughing, crying, and watching different types of movies and TV programs, all may affect your child.

The sensitive, sensible parent observing a regularly occurring reaction to these factors should discuss these findings with his physician or allergist. Together they may be able to devise a plan by which the child would become aware of their findings. They should then proceed toward developing a self-containing role for the child, so that he may become aware of his approximate threshold level in each area. This would permit his continued involvement in the activity to a degree well below his maximum tolerance level.

How To Cope With Asthma

Locate the Offending Allergen

Allow the physician to take tests to determine what your child is allergic to, and to establish a program of desensitization, medication, and other required aspects of treatment. Follow the medical regimen which he establishes. Your allergist can generally diagnose and detect some of the specific offenders. A number of tests are utilized in allergy investigation. Skin testing, an excellent diagnostic method, is done by injecting diluted solutions of suspected allergens under the surface of the patient's skin. The hypersensitive person generally reacts by producing an itchy hive. The nonhypersensitive person usually shows no reaction.

The doctor can often suggest suitable substitutes for things that your child is sensitive to. For example, cotton or synthetic fibers may replace animal products, goat's milk can take the place of cow's milk, and so on.

You perhaps even better than the doctor, can at times help to determine substances which bother your child. Bring these to the attention of your doctor. The doctor may suggest what to stay away from, or give the child desensitization injections to build resistance against the offending allergens.

Desensitization

Since the asthmatic often reacts to certain foods, pollens, or chemicals, the allergist attempts to ascertain which substances cause these allergic reactions. He then proceeds to desensitize the patient by injecting him with an extract of the substance that he is allergic to. Antibodies thus form in the blood which can neutralize the reaction to the allergens to which the child was formerly sensitive. The allergist may include innoculations for pollen, or house dust, animal dander, or other substances, to help build resistance to these things. In addition he may suggest air filters or air conditioning for your house, or make other suggestions for making life easier.

Avoid Offending Allergens

Prevention is a sensible way of stemming attacks. Avoid, or keep your distance from things that are known to irritate or cause wheezing. If dust is one of the offenders, avoid attics and storerooms. Cover mattresses and pillows with allergen-proof plastics or other materials. Use washable blankets and avoid dust catchers such as carpets, drapes, and upholstered furniture. If mildew or mold is an offender, avoid damp basements, and find out how to keep storage areas dry.

If sensitivity exists to feathers, fur, or animal dander, avoid a pet canary, parakeet, dog, cat, or rabbit. Also avoid fur gloves, woolens, and feather pillows. As a precaution, make certain that synthetic or cotton blankets, bedspreads, curtains, mattress covers, and pillows are washable.

Always avoid smoking, chemicals, paints, and insecticides. Avoid fumes, and try to stay away from smoke-filled rooms and from people who are smoking. Avoid weeds and uncut fields.

Temperature Changes and Sensitivity to Physical Factors

If abrupt changes in weather affect your child, do not have him go from heated areas into the cold, or from a warm climate immediately into an air-conditioned room. If he is bothered by strong drafts, suggest that he stay out of them or dress appropriately.

Notice how he is affected by cola, coffee, or alcoholic beverages. Do they stimulate mucus secretions?

Be sensitive not only to physical irritants, but to overwork, overtiredness, and to emotional upset. The chances are that your child's resistance to allergens or irritants will be lowered when he is tired or disturbed.

Think over what he may be allergic to. When an allergic respiratory symptom occurs, try to connect the symptom with a particular food, or with some other irritant which the child was exposed to before the onset of the symptom. Think of all possible offenders: consider foods, hair sprays, deodorants, cosmetics, perfumes, headache powders and tranquilizers. Try to keep your child away from the suspected offenders for several days and see what happens. Tell your doctor about it if allergic symptoms occur after he is exposed to the substance again.

Relating to Your Child

Try to get to know your child better, and to understand his feelings. Encourage him to talk things over, to discuss his fears, his doubts, his anxieties, and his apprehensions. Provide opportunities for him to talk. A suitable time might be at meals or before bedtime. Don't limit your conversations to his illness; rather try to immerse yourself in the world of the child, considering his feelings about friends, school, teachers, and experiences.

Avoid being overly punitive! Allow the expression of feelings freely. It is not necessary for you to react or respond or have an answer for everything that your child brings up. Be attentive! Don't cut your child's conversation short!

Be Observant

Try to be cognizant of how your child acts with others. Observe how he gets along with his brothers, sisters, and friends. Try to find out what makes him happy and what makes him sad, what he thinks of himself and of others, and what others think of him.

Reflect with him on some of your observations during rap sessions. Encourage him to verbalize by offering an opening such as, "I see that you are annoyed by _____. Let's talk about it." Or begin with, "You seem very happy today; something nice must have happened. Tell me about it." It might be a worthwhile investment to acquire a copy of *Parent Effectiveness Training* by Thomas Gordon.[88] Dr. Gordon devotes several chapters to methods and suggestions for establishing communication between parents and children.

Limits

After you've shared your observations and findings with your physician, discussed your child's physical condition—including whether he is able to participate in gym, sports, running, and various games—and determined his physical capabilities, place only the minimum restrictions necessary upon him.

Tolerance Level

Observe how your child fares under the physician's suggested regimen and see what his tolerance threshold is. As indicated, you can determine this through simple observation. How much running, jumping, or swimming is required before wheezing or other features preliminary to an asthmatic attack begin to develop? Encourage your child to become aware of these symptoms so that he can become self-regulating, participating and enjoying involvement in favored activities, but stopping before he exceeds his tolerance limit.

Try to avoid having your child interpret these limitations as punishment. Encourage him rather to participate in activities which he enjoys. For example, if he likes to ride his bike, and you have observed that the wheezing begins after he does so, encourage him to reduce his riding time and to follow it with an activity which is less demanding physically.

Have available a toy box with quiet games such as checkers and chess, picture puzzles, Monopoly, comic books, and water colors, so that the child can shift gears from a physically taxing to a less demanding activity when he reaches his tolerance level without feeling that he is being deprived of a good time, or that he is being punished by having his active play time shortened. If possible, arrange for him to share this next quiet activity with a friend, so that he does not feel isolated socially.

Sleep and Rest

How much sleep or rest does your child require? The chances are that he is more susceptible to an attack, as many children are, when he is overtired, or has received insufficient rest or sleep. Encourage him to obtain the rest and relaxation necessary to function at his maximum effectiveness. If your child is of preschool age, consider the importance of a regular nap.

Help the child develop an interest in such nontaxing activities as hobbies, reading, and in the arts of conversation and communication. Encourage him to simmer down and unwind if he has had a physically or emotionally exhausting day. Participate with him if you can or encourage him to play with other children; read to him from a favorite book, or play a quiet game with him.

Be Supportive

Accept your child for what he is, and encourage him to function to the best of his abilities on his own level. This means that goals and expectations for him must be compatible with his talents, and not with unrealistic notions you or someone else may have. Bear in mind that unrealistic expectations which cannot be fulfilled, will cause feelings of fright and guilt, and can contribute to the creation of stress which you are trying to avoid.

Try to understand what your child's goals are. You can assist your child by helping him develop better insights into himself, his talents, and his skills and capabilities.

Build upon his strengths. If he exhibits interests and capabilities in specific areas, encourage him to try these. Motivate interest in new areas, and introduce him to new skills periodically to help him acquire a sense of accomplishment and growth. But don't push him beyond his capacity; allow him to progress at his own speed and on his own level. Letting him move at his own pace will help him achieve a measure of independence. Don't hold on to the apron strings too tightly.

Treat Him Like a Normal Child

Don't view your child as fragile.

While maintaining a sympathetic understanding of his limitations, avoid placing upon him unnecessary restrictions on movement and activity beyond those established by his physician, and by the tolerance levels you have set. Focus on your child's positive abilities and attributes. Identify his strengths. As the old song goes, try to "accentuate the positive, and eliminate the negative." To support and build is more productive and rewarding for your child's health than nagging. Try to see the healthy part of his personality, and to conduct as normal a routine for your family and your child as possible.

Don't Manipulate

Just as you would have your child avoid manipulating you through his illness, be careful about similarly manipulating him to comply with your needs and expectations. Try to gain as much insight as possible into yourself and your family's dynamics, and to understand how your child's illness affects you and your family. Most people need professional help from a reputable pyschologist, social worker, or psychiatrist to fully understand their child's and their own emotional states and the possible interrelationship and effect of both on his condition. Our bias, as you are aware by now, is for this to take place in a small social or therapy group where your youngster can associate with others his age and condition, and where you too can share with parents like yourself your frustrations, your feelings of love and anger, guilt and despair. Cooperate with your therapist, and understand that there may be some rough going in the process. Be open and cooperative, and avoid sabotaging the therapy.

Special Interests

Avoid comparing your child with other children in or outside your family. Encourage him to develop social relationships with other youngsters. Each child needs a special friend. A loyal pal is especially needed when one is under the weather. A good place to cultivate social contacts is at the local Y, community center, or youth group at your place of worship. Special interest groups concerned with art, photography, newspaper, reporting, drama, crafts, and other skills in which the youngster is interested and in which he can achieve satisfying results from his efforts and experiences, are particularly desirable.

Set up a hobby corner, equip it with nonallergenic clay and finger paints, and encourage your child to use these to get rid of his frustrations and pent-up feelings. A punching bag may serve a similar purpose.

If the child is allergic to pets and animals consider, perhaps, a fish tank, or autograph, coin, or stamp collecting, or gardening (if he is not allergic to pollens and dust). Choose an activity in which he can simultaneously cultivate a feeling of responsibility and achieve satisfaction and reward.

Avoid allergic foods and contact with other allergenic substances. Instead, where possible, provide alternatives, cookies, and food treats which can satisfy his needs and not set him too far apart from his nonallergenic friends.

How to Control Anxiety and Stress

As we have pointed out, a common question running through each stage of man's development is one of how to cope; how to adjust our yearnings, needs, and strivings, with the realities of given situations to minimize the impact of stressors on both our physical and emotional health.

Psychologists Jerome Singer and David Glass (authors of *Urban Stress*), believe that "feelings of control" can often help people better tolerate and reduce the effects of stress. Since everybody lives in a stressful environment at one time or another, it is useful, they suggest, "to try to develop some general approaches" to combat it.[89]

Their recommendations include the following, which you might try to utilize yourself and adapt for use by your child:

1. *Relax.* "It is likely that you are going to adapt to stresses anyhow, and there is nothing to be gained by working yourself up."
2. *Place Stress In a Favorable Context.* "If you can convince yourself that the source of stress is useful or 'necessary,' " they advise, "you will have less or no stress afterwards."
3. *Regularize Your Environment.* "The same stressors will be less harmful if they occur predictably." Behaviorists feel that a person can often make stress more predictable "by arranging his schedule to fit the occurrences of the stress."
4. *Arrange for Control.* "Try to arrange situations so that you have the possibilities of controlling the stress," Singer and

Glass recommend, "even though you may choose not to exercise this control." This may be an effective way to "minimize its [stress'] consequences."

5. *Develop Sensitivity to Long-Term Perspectives.* Develop a philosophy that "sometimes moderate stress must be endured in order to avoid ultimate disaster.⁹⁰

Some Additional Suggestions for Asthmatics

Try to incorporate some of the following into your life philosophy:

—When possible, try to avoid situations, activities, or events which tend to precipitate anger. Since even pleasant events which stimulate or excite can be stressful, keep these within bounds. Remember that the hormone balance can become upset by emotional changes, good or bad.

—Try to reduce the frequency of change. Do not get involved in too many new projects or changes at once. If you have to introduce changes—of residence, job, friends, experiences—try to take them slowly, and to limit them to one at a time.

Consider relaxation as an important part of your life. Build it into your schedule, and try to find time to take it easy.

—Slow down and enjoy. Take the time to look at the world around you, to read, to think, to dream, to discover some of nature's beauties.

—Eat and drink more slowly. Enjoy your food. Don't gulp!

—Try to be yourself more often. Stop responding the way others expect you to respond, and try to do things that *you* like to do, the way you want.

—Be accepting of yourself—of your strengths as well as your limitations. Do not be too disappointed with yourself! No one is perfect.

—Seek out nice people to socialize and interact with. It will help you to get your mind off yourself. Avoid people who anger or annoy you.

—Try to alternate interests and hobbies.

—Take breaks from strenuous or taxing activities that build up pressure or tension.

Change May Be Possible, But Don't Expect Miracles

With a little give and a great deal of understanding and effort, it may be possible to determine how emotional and psychological factors operate in tandem with physical factors for you or your child. When this occurs, and it becomes possible to relieve some of the pressures precipitating or aggravating the condition, it is hoped the strains can be diffused and the vicious circle of the disease's cause and consequence broken.

Though this is within the realm of possibility, it is wise to bear in mind that notwithstanding yours, your physician's and your therapist's best efforts, your child's illness may not totally disappear. If and when an attack occurs, keep your wits about you; utilize the medications and procedures recommended by your physician. Continue to be understanding and sympathetic, though not rewarding, about the illness. This latter point is worth thinking about, since the child who receives gifts and favored treatment when he is ill may subtly be encouraged to continue his illness pattern.

Continue making your best efforts to think and act positively!

12

EXERCISES TO STRENGTHEN THE MUSCLES OF RESPIRATION AND TO HELP CLEAR THE AIRWAYS

Strengthening the Muscles of Respiration

What follows is a series of exercises to strengthen the scapula (muscles of respiration), the lower intercostals, and the diaphragm, with the primary purpose to "mobilize the chest." In addition to correcting posture, these activities can help correct breathing and increase vital pulmonary capacity. They can also, through increased competence in respiration and expiration, teach breath control and inspire confidence in a youngster's ability to abort or control an attack. Check the suitability of each with your doctor.

Breathing in, inspiration, is an act that we perform without undo concern or effort. Formal, conscious breathing entails taking about a pint of air into the lungs, and pushing out, or expiring, about the same amount. The amount of air which we can take in each time we breathe depends upon the amount which has been let out. The more a person is able to let out, the more fresh air he can let in. In order to aerate properly, it is important for the child to learn how to expel or push the maximum amount of air out of his lungs.

A good way to begin is through exercises in pursed-lip breathing. The child is encouraged first to expire in order to push out as much air as he normally can. He then purses his lips as if to whistle silently and keeps forcing air out until he feels that his diaphragm is as far up in his chest as it can go. Then he takes as deep a breath as he can through his nose until he can feel the diaphragm bellowing out, and lets the air out gently, without force.

Other Breathing Exercises

The exercises explained in this section are intended to help train the chest and stomach muscles to assist in breathing.
Try to do your exercises when you get up, before you eat, and/or before bedtime.

Make yourself comfortable! Remove tight clothing. Be sure that your breathing passages are clear. Don't hurry your exercises, and rest when necessary. Try to relax!

Take a deep breath, and then exhale slowly. Breathing too fast puts an unnecessary burden on your lungs.

The following exercises have been adapted from a list prepared by the Physical Fitness Center for Asthmatic Children:[91]

1. *Circle*: Hold arms out at shoulder level. Turn circles in one direction 10 times, then reverse 10 times.
2. *The Squeezer*: Stand erect. Squeeze shoulders back and attempt to touch elbows behind you 10 times.
3. *The Roller*: Roll both shoulders up toward your ears and circle clockwise 5 times. Then reverse direction and circle 5 times.

4. *Standing Breathing Exercise*: Stand erect and inhale to the count of two, then exhale to the count of 6 or 8 by hissing out.

5. *Trunk Twist*: Standing straight with your arms at your sides, perpendicular to your body, twist your trunk toward your left side 10 times; then reverse your direction and twist your trunk to the right side 10 times.

6. *Toe Touch*: Stand erect with feet slightly apart. Touch your left hand to your right toe 10 times, then your right hand to your left toe 10 times.

7. *Squat*: Place your hands on your hips (keep your back straight) and hiss air out while squatting down. Inhale deeply while rising up. Repeat 10 times.

8. *Push-ups*: Lie face down on floor. Place hands on floor palms-down at shoulder level. Attempt to raise body while supporting weight on arms. (Try to keep body straight). Repeat several times.

9. *Sit-ups*: Sit on the floor. Clasp hands in back of head. Lean back slowly until your head touches floor. Inhale while doing so. Then sit up slowly. Exhale by hissing on the way up. Repeat several times.

10. *Breathing Exercises Lying Down*: Lie on your back. Place a five pound weight on your chest. Breathe with your diaphragm.

NOTES

1. Young, Patrick. "Asthma and Allergies, An Optimistic Future." U.S. Department of Health and Human Services, Publication Health Services, National Institute of Health, NIH Publication No. 80-388, March, 1980, 16.
2. Children's Bureau Survey, United States Department of Health, Education, and Welfare. Publication 72-281, 1972, Table 1. "of all allergic conditions, asthma is usually considered the most serious. Asthma is the leading cause of active limitation in people under 17 years of age in the United States." Additional source: NCHS-PHS, series 10, #61.
3. Pappel, Catherine, and Rothman, Beulah. Social Group Work Models. *Social Work with Groups*. Adelphi School of Social Work. 1969, 1, (1).
4. For a fuller description of Allergic Asthma, see *Textbook of Medicine*, edited by Beeson, Paul B., and Walsh McDermott, James B. Wyngaarden, 15th Edition, Philadelphia, Saunders, 1979, 956ff.
5. Adapted from *Allergic Diseases,* Allergy Foundation of America, New York, N. Y. 19.
6. See Psychodynamics of Asthma. *Journal of Asthma Research* 1965, 3:1, 12.
7. Lask, Aaron. *Asthma, Attitude, and Milieu.* Philadelphia, Lippincott, 1966, 193 ff.

147

8. Alcock, T. Some Personality Characteristics of Asthmatic Children, *British Journal of Medical Psychology,* 1960, *33,* 133-146.
9. Turner, C. H. Asthma in Children: Psychogenic Aspects. *North Carolina Medical Journal,* 1961, *22,* 517-522.
10. Little, S. W., and Cohen, L. D. Goal Setting Behavior of Asthmatic Children and Their Mothers for Them. *Journal of Personality,* 1951, *19,* 376-394.
11. Rogerson, C. H. Psychological Factors in Asthma-Prurigo. *Quarterly Journal of Medicine,* 1937, *6,* 367-394.
12. Gillespie, R. D. Psychological Factors in Asthma. *British Medical Journal,* 1936, *1,* 1285-1289.
13. Leigh, David, and Lovett, D. Asthma and Psychosis. *Journal of Mental Science,* 1953, *99,* 489-496.
14. Little, S. W. and Cohen, L. D. Ibid, 100.
15. Mitchel, A. J., Frost, L., and Marx, R. Emotional Aspects of Pediatric Allergy-The Role of the Mother-Child Relationship. *Annals of Allergy,* 1953, *11,* 744 ff.
16. Sperling, Melita, Asthma in Children, An Evaluation of Concepts and Therapies. *Journal of American Academy of Child Psychiatry,* 1968, *7,* 44-58.
17. French, Thomas, and Alexander, Frank. Psychogenic Factors in Bronchial Asthma. *Psychomatic Medicine,* 1941, *4,* (1). Monograph IV Part I and II Washington, D. C.; National Research Council.
18. Miller, H., and Baruch, D., Emotional Problems of Childhood and their Relationship to Asthma. *American Journal of Diseases of Children,* 1957, *93,* 242.
19. Miller and Baruch, Ibid.
20. Peshkin, M. Murray, and Abraham Harold. The Treatment of Institutionalized Children with Intractable Asthma. *Connecticut Medicine,* 1960, *24,* (166), 43-44.
21. Maurer, Endre, The Child with Asthma. An Assessment of Relative Importance of Emotional Factors. *Journal of Asthma Research,* 1965, 3:25-79.
22. Abramson, Harold. Evaluation of Maternal Rejection Theory in Allergy. *Annals of Allergy,* 1954, 12:129-140.
23. McGovern, John and Knight, James. A. *Allergy and Human Emotions.* Springfield, Illinois, Thomas, 1967, 18ff.
24. Strecker, Edward, H. Appel, Kenneth, and Appel, John. *Discovering Ourselves. A View of the Human Mind and How It Works.* New York: Macmillan, 1960, 113-160.
25. Steincron, Peter. *You Live as You Breathe.* New York: McKay, 1967, 21.
26. Strecker, E., Appel, K. and Appel, J. Ibid, 24.
27. McGladshan, Alan. Breakfast Breakthrough. *The Lancet,* October 9, 1971, 812.
28. Thomas, W. I. Personality Links to Cancer, Heart Disease. *Sci-*

ence News, 1975, *108*, 182.

29. Haugen, G. B., and Dixon, H. H., and Dickel, H. A. *A Therapy for Anxiety, Tension Reactions.* New York: Macmillan, 1963.
30. Thomas, W. I. Ibid.
31. Holmes, Thomas, and Rahe, Richard. The Social Readjustment Rating Scale. *Journal of Psychosomatic Research*, 1967, 11:213-218.
32. Holmes, T. and Rahe, R. Ibid.
33. Holmes, Thomas, and Minoru, Masuda. *Psychology Today*, April 1972, Del Mar, CA.
34. Holmes, T., and Rahe, R. Ibid.
35. Holmes, T., and Rahe, R. Ibid.
36. Lewis, Howard, and Lewis, Martha, E. *Psychosomatics—How Your Emotions Can Damage your Health.* New York, Viking Press, 1972.
37. Cannon, Walter, B. *The Wisdom of the Body and Flight or Fight. Stress, Our Friend, Our Foe, Blueprint for Health*, Chicago, Illinois, Blue Cross Association, 1974, *25*:1.
38. Selye, Hans. *Stress of Life.* New York: McGraw Hill, 1976, 171ff.
39. Selye. Ibid.
40. Harris, M. C. Is There a Specific Emotional Pattern In Allergic Disease? *Annals of Allergy*, 1955, *13*, 654-661.
41. Friedman, Meyer, and Rosenman, Roy. *Type A Behavior and Your Heart.* New York: Knopf, 1974.
42. Rose, Alan. Emotion and Rheumatoid Arthritis. *Medical World News*, April, 1972.
43. Weiner, H., Thaler, M. Emotion and Duodenal Ulcer. *Psychosomatic Medicine*, 1957, *19*, 1.
44. Pinkerton, Philip, Childhood Asthma. *British Journal of Hospital Medicine*, September, 1971, *6*, 331-338.
45. Pearson, Bruce. Conference at Maudsley Hospital. London, April, 1955. *Journal of Psychosomatic Research*, 1956, *1*:(169).
46. Schwab, John J. *Handbook of Psychiatric Consultation.* New York: Appleton Centry Crofts, 1969, 3.
47. Lewin, Kurt. *Field Theory in Social Science: Selected Theoretical Papers.* New York: Harper Row, 1951.
48. Schwab, J. Ibid, 11ff.
49. Schwab, J. Ibid.
50. Schwab, J. Ibid.
51. Peshkin, M. Murray. Asthma in Children. Role of Environment in the Treatment of Selected Group of Cases. *American Journal of Diseases of Children*, 1930, *39*, 774-781.
52. Peshkin, M. Murray. Ibid. 44.
53. Peshkin, M. Murray. Intractable Asthma of Childhood. Rehabilitation at the Institutional Level—With a Follow-up of 150 cases. *International Archives of Allergy*, 1959, 15:91-112.
54. Peshkin, M. Murray. Ibid.
55. Also see Peshkin, M. Murray. Significance of Time Lag and At-

tack Stages of Asthma. *Journal of Asthma Research*, 1968, *6*, (1), 5-11.

56. Long, R. T.; Lamont, H. H.; Whipple, Bandler, Blom, J. E.; Burgen, L., Jessner. A Psychosomatic Study of Allergic and Emotional Factors in Children With Asthma. *American Journal of Psychiatry*, 1958, *114*, 890-899.

57. Purcell, Kenneth. The Effect on Asthma in Children of Experimental Separation From the Family. *Psychosomatic Medicine*, 1969, *3*, 144-164.

58. Falliers, Constantine J. Treatment of Asthma in a Residential Center - A Fifteen Year Study. *Annals of Allergy*, 28:513-521.

59. Peshkin, M. Murray. The Role of Residential Asthma Centers for Children With Intractable Asthma. *Journal of Asthma Research*, 1968, 6:(2), 66.

60. Sperling. Ibid, 46.

61. Parents/Children—Where Disturbed Parents Can Learn to Live Together. *New York Times*, February 7, 1975, 37.

62. Luparello, Thomas. Psychological Factors and Laboratory Models for Investigation of Bronchial Asthma. *New York State Journal of Medicine*, September, 15, 1971, 2161-2165.

63. Tuft, H. S. The Development and Management of Intractable Asthma in Childhood. *American Journal of Disabled Child*, 1957, *93*, 251.

64. Purcell, Kenneth, Bernstein, Lewis, and Bukantz, Samuel. A Preliminary Comparison of Rapidly Remitting and Persistently Steroid Dependent Asthmatic Children. *Psychosomatic Medicine*, 1961, 23:4, 305-310.

65. Krakelien, J. Asthma Research in Children's Department. Karolinska Sjokhuset. *Journal of Asthma Research*, 1968, *6*, (2) 75.

66. Wohl, Theodore H. The Group Approach to the Asthmatic Child and Family. *Journal of Asthma Research*, 1967, *4* (4) 238.

67. Wohl, Ibid.

68. Ghory, Joseph. The Short Term Patient in a Convalescent Hospital Asthma Program. *Journal of Asthma Research*, 1966, 3.3 243ff.

69. Israel Ministry of Health Survey, 1975. Also see Table 1 *Allergy Research—an Introduction*, Publication 19 #72-281, 1972 NIH, U.S. Dept. of HEW.

70. Vintner, Robert. *Social Work, 19*:15.

71. Dreikuss, Rudolf. Group Psychotherapy From the Point of View of Adlerian Psychology. *In Group Therapy Today—Styles, Methods and Techniques*, Hendrik Ruitenbeck, ed. Atherton Press, 1969, 73.

72. Dreikuss, R. Ibid.

73. Slavson, S. R. *Early Experiments With Group Psychology*, in Hendrik Ruitenbeck, Ibid, 36ff.

74. Dreikuss, R. Ibid, 68.

75. Slavson, S. R. Ibid, 38.

76. Slavson, S. R. Ibid, 40.
77. Yalom, Irving. *The Theory and Practice of Group Psychotherapy.* New York: Basic, 1970, 354ff.
78. Horney, Karen. *Neurosis and Human Growth: The Struggle Toward Self-Realization.* New York: Norton, 1950, 351.
79. Argyris, C. Conditions for Competence Acquisition and Therapy. *Journal of Applied Behavioral Sciences,* 1968, *4*, 147-179.
80. Frank, Jerome. Training and Therapy. In L. P. Bradford, J. R. Gibb, and K. D. Benne. *Group Therapy and Laboratory Method: Innovation in Education.* New York: Wiley, 1964.
81. Yalom. Ibid.
82. Rogers, Carl. On Becoming a Person. *A Therapist's View of Psychotherapy.* Boston: Houghton Mifflin, 1961, 64.
83. Rogers, C. Ibid
84. Rogers, C. Ibid
85. Rogers, C. Ibid
86. Rogers, C. Ibid
87. Salk, Lee. Growing Up Mentally Fit. *Stress,* 1974, *25*, (1) 18-25.
88. Gordon, Thomas. *P.E.T.—Parent Effectiveness Training.* 88. Gordon, York: Widen, 1970, 140.
89. Singer, Jerome, and Glass, David. Making Your World More Livable. *Stress,* 1974, *25*, 59.
90. Singer, p. 65.
91. Exercises Courtesy Physical Fitness Center for Asthmatic Children, prepared by the Allergy Foundation of America, New York Infirmary, New York, N. Y.

REFERENCES

Abramson, Harold. Evaluation of the Maternal Rejection Theory in Allergy. *Annals of Allergy*, 1954, 12:129-140.

Alcock, T. Some Personality Characteristics of Asthmatic Children. *British Journal of Medical Psychology*, 1960, (33), 133-146.

Alexander, A. B., Miklich, D. R. and Hershkoff, H. The Immediate Effects of Systematic Relaxation Training on Peak Expiratory Flow Rates in Asthmatic Children. *Psychosomatic Medicine*, 1972, 34:388-394.

Alexander, F. G., and Selasnick, S. T. *The History of Psychiatry.* New York: Harper & Row, 1966.

Allergic Diseases. New York: Allergy Foundation of America, 19.

Argyris, C. Conditions for Competence Acquisition and Therapy. *Journal of Applied Behavioral Sciences*, 1968, *4*, 147-179.

Block, J. H., E. Harvey, P. H. Jenning, and E. Simpson. Clinicians' Conceptions of the Asthmatogenic Mother. *Archives of General Psychiatry*, 1966, 15:610-618.

Cannon, Walter, B. *The Wisdom of the Body and Flight or Fight.* New York, Norton, 1932.

Coleman, Harris, M., and Shivel, Norman. *All About Allergy.* Englewood Cliffs, N. J.: Prentice-Hall, 1969.

De Gara, Paul F. Early Treatment of Allergy-Does the Child Outgrow It? *Journal of Asthma Research*, 1966, *3*, (3), 181-184.

Dreiskuss, Rudolf. Group Psychotherapy From the Point of View of Adlerian Psychology. In *Group Therapy Today. Styles, Methods and Techniques.* Henricke Ruitenbeck, Ed. New York: Atherton Press, 1969, 73.

Falliers, Constantine, J. Treatment of Asthma in a Residential Center—a Fifteen Year Study. *Annals of Allergy,* 28:513-521.

Frank, Jerome. Training and Therapy. in L. P. Bradford, J. R. Gibb, and K. D. Benne, (eds.) *Group Therapy and Laboratory Method: Innovation in Education.* New York: Wiley, 1964.

French, Thomas M., and Alexander, Frank. Psychogenic Factors in Bronchial Asthma. *Psychosomatic Medicine*, 1941, *4* (1). Monograph IV, Volume 2, Part I and II, Washington, D.C.: National Research Council.

Friedman, Meyer, and Rosenman, Roy. *Type A Behavior and Your Heart.* New York: Knopf, 1974.

Gillespie, R. D. Psychological Factors in Asthma. *British Medical Journal*, 1936, *1*, 1285-1289.

Glasberg, H. M., P.M. Bromberg, M. Stein, and T. J. Luparello. A Personality Study of Asthmatic Patients. *Journal of Psychosomatic Research*, 1969, 13:197-204.

Goldberg, E. L., and G. W. Constock. Life Events and Subsequent Illness. *American Journal of Epidemiology*, 1976, 104:146-158.

Gordon, Thomas. *P.E.T.—Parent Effectiveness Training.* New York: Widen, 1970.

Grinker, R. R. The Psychosomatic Aspects of Anxiety. *Anxiety and Behavior*, ed. C. D. Spielberger, New York: Academic Press, 1966.

Harris, M. C. Is There a Specific Emotional Pattern in Allergic Disease? *Annals of Allergy*, 1955, 13, 654-661.

Haugen, G. B., Dixon, H.H., and Dickel, H. A. *A Theory for Anxiety, Tension Reaction.* New York: Macmillan, 1963.

Herbert, M., R. Glick, and H. Black. Olfactory Precipitation of Bronchial Asthma. *Journal Psychosomatic Research*, 1967, 11:195-202.

Hinkle, L. E. Ecological Observations of the Relation of Physical Illness, Mental Illness and the Social Environment. *Psychosomatic Medicine*, 1961, *23*, 289.

Holmes, T. H., and M. Masuda. Life Change and Illness Susceptibility. *Stressful Life Events: Their Nature and Effects*, ed. B. S. and B. P. Dohrenwend, New York: Wiley, 1974.

Horney, Karen. *Neurosis and Human Growth: The Struggle Toward Self-Realization.* New York: W. W. Norton, 1950, 351.

Jenkins, C. D., R. H. Rosenman, and M. Friedman. Development of an Objective Psychological Test for the Determination of the Coronary-Prone Behavior Pattern of Employed Men. *Journal of Chronic Diseases*, 1967, 20:371-379.

Kellner, R. Psychotherapy in Psychosomatic Disorders. *Archives of General Psychiatry*, 1975 32:1021-28.

Knapp, P. H., A. A. Mathe, and L. Vachon. Psychosomatic Aspects of Bronchial Asthma. *Bronchial Asthma, Its Nature and Management*, ed. E. B. Weis and M. S. Segal. Boston: Little, Brown, 1976.

Krakelien, J. Asthma Research in Children's Department. Karolinska Sjukhuset. *Journal of Asthma Research*, 1968, *6* (2), 75.

Lask, Aaron. *Asthma, Attitude and Milieu.* Philadelphia: Lippincott, 1966, 193. ff.

Liebman, R., S. Minuchin, and L. Baker. The Use of Structural Family Therapy in the Treatment of Intractable Asthma. *American Journal of Psychiatry*, 1974, 131, no. 5:535-540.

Leigh, David, and Lovett, D., Asthma and Psychosis. *Journal of Mental Science*, 1953, *99*, 484-496.

Lewin, Kurt. *Field Theory in Social Science: Selected Theoretical Papers.* New York: Harper and Row, 1951.

Lewis, Howard R., and Lewis, Martha E. *Psychosomatics—How Your Emotions Can Damage Your Health.* New York: Viking, 1972.

Little, S. W., and Cohen, L. D. Goal-Setting Behavior of Asthmatic Children and Their Mothers for Them. *Journal of Personality*, 1951, *19*, 376-394.

Long, R. T., Lamont, J.H., Whipple, B., Bandler, L., Blom, J., Burgen, L., and Jessner, L. A. Psychosomatic Study of Allergic and Emotional Factors in Children with Asthma. *American Journal of Psychiatry*, 1958, *114*, 890-899.

Luparello, Thomas. Psychological Factors and Laboratory Models for Investigation of Bronchial Asthma. *New York State Journal of Medicine*, September 15, 1971, 2161-2165.

Mathe, A. A., and Knapp, P.H., Emotional and Adrenal Reactions to Stress in Bronchial Asthma. *Psychosomatic Medicine*, 1971, 33:323-340.

Maurer, Endre. The Child with Asthma, An Assessment of Relative Importance of Emotional Factors. *Journal of Asthma Research*. 1965, *3*, 25-79.

McGlashan, Alan. Breakfast Breakthrough. *The Lancet*, October 9, 1971, 812.

McGovern, John and Knight, James, A. *Allergy and Human Emotions.* Springfield, Illinois: Thomas, 1967, 18 ff.

McKenzie, J. N. The Production of "Rose Asthma" by an Artificial Rose. *American Journal of Medical Science*, 1886, 91:45-57.

Miller, H., and Baruch, Dorothy. Emotional Problems of Childhood and Their Relationship to Asthma. *American Journal of Diseases of Children*, 1957, *93*, 242.

Miller, H. and D. W. Baruch, Psychosomatic Studies of Children with Allergic Manifestations: Maternal Rejection: A Study of Sixty-three cases. *Psychosomatic Medicine*, 1948, 10:275-278.

Mitchel, A. J., Frost, L., and Marx, R. Emotional Aspects of Pediatric Allergy. The Role of the Mother-Child Relationship. *Annals of Allergy*, 1953, *11*, 744ff.

Moore, Norah. Behavior Therapy in Bronchial Asthma. A Controlled Study. *Journal of Psychosomatic Research* 1965, *9*, 257-276.

Oken, Donald, M.D. Stress, Our Friend, Our Foe, in Stress. *Blue Print for Health*, 1974, Blue Cross Association, Chicago, Illinois, *25*, (1).

Pappel, Catherine and Rothman, Beulah, Social Group Work Models. *Social Work with Groups*, Adelphi School of Social Work. 1969, 1, (1).

Pearson, Bruce. Conference at Maudsley Hospital, London, April 1955. *Journal of Psychosomatic Research*, 1956, *1*, (169).

Peshkin, M. Murray. Asthma in Children. Role of Environment in the Treatment of a Selected Group of Cases. *American Journal of Dis-*

eases of Children, 1930, *39*, 774-781.

Peshkin, M. Murray. Significance of Time Lag and Attack Stages of Asthma. *Journal of Asthma Research*, 1968, *6*, (1), 5-11.

Peshkin, M. Murray. The Role of Residential Asthma Centers for Children with Intractable Asthma. *Journal of Asthma Research*, 1968, *6*, (2).

Peshkin, M. Murray, and Abraham, Harold. The Treatment of Institutionalized Children with Intractable Asthma. *Connecticut Medicine*, 1960, *24*, (166), 43-44.

Pinkerton, Philip. Childhood Asthma. *British Journal of Hospital Medicine*, September 1971, *6*, 331-338.

Purcell, K., L., Bernstein, and Bukantz, S. A Preliminary Comparison of Rapidly Remitting and Persistently "Steroid-Dependent" Asthmatic Children. *Psychosomatic Medicine*, 1961, 23:4, 305-310.

Rahe, R. H. Subjects' Recent Life Changes and Their Near Future Illness Reports. *Annals of Clinical Research*, 1973, 4:1-16.

Rahe, R. H., J. L. Mahan, Jr., and R. J. Arthur. Prediction of Near-Future Health Change From Subjects' Preceding Life Changes. *Journal of Psychosomatic Research*, 1970, 14:401-406.

Rogers, Carl. A Theory of Therapy, Personality and Interpersonal Relationships. In S. Koch (ed.) *Psychology: A Study of Science* (Vol. 3) New York; McGraw-Hill, 1959, 184-256.

Rogers, Carl. *On Becoming a Person. A Therapist's View of Psychosomatic Research*, 1970, 14:401-406.

Rogers, Carl. A Theory of Therapy, Personality and Interpersonal Relationships. In S. Koch. (ed.) *Psychology: A Study of Science* (Vol. 3) New York: McGraw-Hill, 1959, 184-256.

Rogers, Carl. On Becoming a Person. *A Therapist's View of Psychotherapy*. Boston: Houghton Mifflin, 1961, 64.

Rogers, Carl. *The Process of the Basic Encounter Group*. La Jolla, Calif.: Western Behavioral Institute, 1966.

Rogerson, C. H. Psychological Factors in Asthma-Prurigo. *Quarterly Journal of Medicine*, 1937, *6*, 367-394.

Ruitenbeck, Hendrik (ed.) *Group Therapy Today—Styles, Methods and Techniques*. New York: Atherton Press, 1969.

Salk, Lee. Growing Up Mentally Fit. *Stress*, 1974, *25*, (1).

Schaffer, Nathan. Atopic Dermatitis in the Older Child. *Journal of Asthma Research*, 1966, 3 (3), 189.

Schneer, H. I. A Psychoanalytic Study of Bronchial Asthma in Children. In *The Asthmatic Child*, New York: Harper and Row, 1963.

Schwab, John J. *Handbook of Psychiatric Consultation*. New York: Appleton Century Crofts, 1969.

Selye, H. The General Adaptation Syndrome and the Diseases of Adaptation. *Journal of Clinical Endocrinology and Metabolism*, 1946, 6:117-230.

Selye, Hans. *Stress of Life*. New York: McGraw-Hill, 1976, 171ff.

Singer, Jerome and Glass, David. Making Your World More Livable. *Stress*, 1974, *25*, 59.

Slavson, S. R. Early Experiments with Group Psychology. In H. Ruitenbeck (ed.) *Group Therapy Today—Style, Methods and Techniques*. New York: Atherton Press, 1969, 36.

Speer, Frederic. *The Management of Childhood Asthma*. Springfield, Ill.: Charles C. Thomas, 1958.

Sperling, Melita. Asthma in Children, An Evaluation of Concepts and Therapies. *Journal of American Academy of Child Psychiatry.*, January 1968, 7, 44-58.

Sperling, M. Psychoanalytic Study of Ulcerative Colitis in Children. *Psychoanalytic Quarterly*, 1946, 15:302-329.

Steincrohn, Peter. *You Live as You Breathe*. New York: McKay, 1967, 21.

Strecher, Edward, Appel, Kenneth, and Appel, John. *Discovering Ourselves—A View of the Human Mind and How It Works*. New York: Macmillan, 1960., 113-160.

Stress, Our Friend, Our Foe, *Blueprint for Health*. 25:1 Blue Cross Association, Chicago, Ill. 1974.

The Ins and Outs of Better Breathing. Elmsford, New York: Boehringer Ingelheim, 1975.

Thomas, Caroline. Personality Links to Cancer, Heart Disease. *Science News*, 1975, *108*, 182.

Tuft, H. S. The Development and Management of Intractable Asthma in Childhood *American Journal Disabled Child*, 1957, 93, 251.

Turner, C. H. Asthma in Children: Psychogenic Aspects. *North Carolina Medical Journal*, 1961, *22*, 517-522.

Vachon, L., and E. S. Rich, Jr. Visceral Learning and Asthma. *Psychosomatic Medicine*, 1976, 38, No. 2:122-130.

Vintner, Robert. *Social Work*, 19, *15*.

Weiner, H. Emotion and Duodenal Ulcer. *Medical World News*, April 1972.

Weiner, H., and Thaler, M. *Psychosomatic Medicine*. 1957, *19*, 1.

Wohl, Theodore, H. The Group Approach to the Asthmatic Child and Family. *Journal of Asthma Research*, 1967, *4* (4), 238.

Yalom, Irving. *The Theory and Practice of Group Psychotherapy*. New York: Basic, 1970, 354ff.

INDEX